Asthma

Asthma

A Clinician's Guide

Margaret Varnell Clark, MS, RN, RRT-NPS

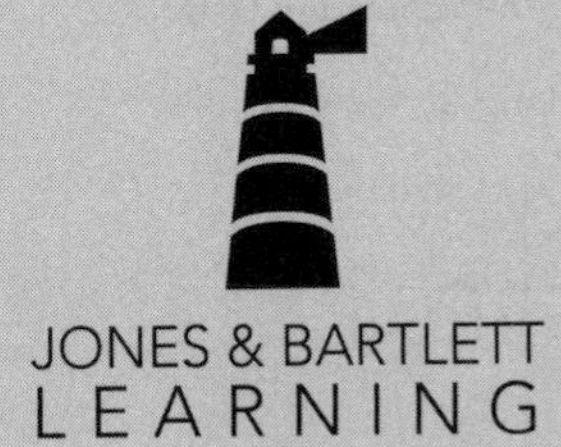

World Headquarters
Jones & Bartlett Learning
40 Tall Pine Drive
Sudbury, MA 01776
978-443-5000
info@jblearning.com
www.jblearning.com

Jones & Bartlett Learning
Canada
6339 Ormindale Way
Mississauga, Ontario L5V 1J2
Canada

Jones & Bartlett Learning
International
Barb House, Barb Mews
London W6 7PA
United Kingdom

Jones & Bartlett Learning books and products are available through most bookstores and online booksellers. To contact Jones & Bartlett Learning directly, call 800-832-0034, fax 978-443-8000, or visit our website, www.jblearning.com.

The author, editor, and publisher have made every effort to provide accurate information. However, they are not responsible for errors, omissions, or for any outcomes related to the use of the contents of this book and take no responsibility for the use of the products and procedures described. Treatments and side effects described in this book may not be applicable to all people; likewise, some people may require a dose or experience a side effect that is not described herein. Drugs and medical devices are discussed that may have limited availability controlled by the Food and Drug Administration (FDA) for use only in a research study or clinical trial. Research, clinical practice, and government regulations often change the accepted standard in this field. When consideration is being given to use of any drug in the clinical setting, the health care provider or reader is responsible for determining FDA status of the drug, reading the package insert, and reviewing prescribing information for the most up-to-date recommendations on dose, precautions, and contraindications, and determining the appropriate usage for the product. This is especially important in the case of drugs that are new or seldom used.

Production Credits
Publisher: David Cella
Associate Editor: Maro Gartside
Editorial Assistant: Teresa Reilly
Production Manager: Julie Champagne Bolduc
Associate Production Editor: Jessica Steele Newfell
Marketing Manager: Grace Richards
Manufacturing and Inventory Control Supervisor: Amy Bacus
Composition: Publishers' Design and Production Services, Inc.
Cover Design: Kristin E. Parker
Cover Image: © Solarseven/Dreamstime.com
Printing and Binding: Malloy, Inc.
Cover Printing: Malloy, Inc.

Library of Congress Cataloging-in-Publication Data
Clark, Margaret Varnell.
Asthma : a clinician's guide / Margaret Varnell Clark.
p. ; cm.
Includes bibliographical references and index.
ISBN 978-0-7637-7854-5
1. Asthma. 2. Asthma—Treatment. I. Title.
[DNLM: 1. Asthma. WF 553 C594a 2011]
RC591.C565 2011
616.2'38—dc22
2010018959

6048

Printed in the United States of America
14 13 12 11 10 10 9 8 7 6 5 4 3 2 1

Brief Contents

Contents

Preface

This book is intended to be a concise resource, making the current guidelines more accessible for healthcare professionals taking care of patients with asthma. More detailed information can be found in the current U.S. guidelines, the National Asthma Education and Prevention Program Expert Panel Report 3: Guidelines for the Diagnosis and Management of Asthma Full Report 2007 from the National Heart, Lung, and Blood Institute. This information is available at:

http://www.nhlbi.nih.gov/guidelines/asthma/asthsumm.pdf.

Acknowledgments

I would like to thank the following individuals for their help and guidance in the development of this book. I couldn't have done it without you! Anthony L. DeWitt, RRT, CRT, JD, FAARC, AANG; Vern Enge, MA; Abigail Goben, MLS; Joan Kohorst, MA, RRT; Doug McIntyre, MS, RRT, FAARC; William M. Stader, CRT, AE-C; and Susan Steinbis, MSN, NP.

About the Author

Margaret Varnell Clark, MS, RN, RRT-NPS, is an award-winning writer and medical editor. She was the Editorial Director for Pulmonary and Critical Care Medicine at Medscape/WebMD from 2004–2009. Prior to this she was the Clinical Coordinator for Respiratory Care, Boston University/Boston Medical Center in Massachusetts. Clark has been a field correspondent for *ADVANCE for Respiratory Care* news magazines since 1990. She is also known for her work with Reuter's Health and PBS television. Clark is the 1996 recipient of the Bird Lifetime Achievement Award given by the American Association of Respiratory Care for her extensive writing on pulmonary medicine. She has served on several boards and committees for the American College of Chest Physicians and has worked and lectured extensively in the United Kingdom, Europe, and Central America.

Reviewers

Marie A. Fenske, EdD, RRT
GateWay Community College
Phoenix, Arizona

Lynda T. Goodfellow, EdD, RRT, AE-C, FAARC
Associate Professor
Georgia State University
Atlanta, Georgia

Donna Johnson, RRT, CPFT, AE-C
Children's Mercy Family Health Partners
Kansas City, Missouri

J. Kenneth Le Jeune, MS, RRT, CPFT
University of Arkansas Community College at Hope
Hope, Arkansas

Mary Martinasek, MPH, RRT
Faculty
Hillsborough Community College
Tampa, Florida

Timothy R. Myers, BS, RRT-NPS
Director of Pediatric Respiratory Care and Procedural Services and Pediatric Heart Center
Rainbow Babies and Children's Hospital
Adjunct Assistant Professor of Pediatrics
Case Western Reserve University
Cleveland, Ohio

Helen Ouellette-Roy, RRT, AE-C
Asthma Education Specialist
Southern Maine Medical Center
Biddeford, Maine

Brian J. Parker, MPH, RRT-NPS, RPFT, AE-C
Chair, Respiratory Care
Baptist College of Health Sciences
Memphis, Tennessee

Candace Ramos, MHA, RRT, AE-C
Senior Education Coordinator
Asthma Management Program
Children's Mercy Family Health Partners
Kansas City, Missouri

Shawna Strickland, MEd, RRT-NPS, AE-C
Respiratory Therapy Program Director and Clinical Assistant Professor
University of Missouri
Columbia, Missouri

Robert D. Tarkowski Jr., MS, RRT-NPS, RPFT
Assistant Professor
Director of Clinical Education
Respiratory Care Program
Gannon University
Erie, Pennsylvania

1 Asthma: A Global Perspective

LEARNING OBJECTIVES

- Discuss the global impact of asthma
- Review the data on hospitalization, costs, mortality, and quality of life for patients with asthma in the United States
- Identify available resources for improving asthma care

KEY WORDS

asthma prevalence
indirect costs
direct costs
EPR-3
quality of life
activities of daily living

The History of Asthma

Asthma is a disease as old as antiquity. The Egyptian Ebers Papyrus found in the 1870s contains prescriptions written in hieroglyphics for asthma that include a mixture of herbs heated on a brick so that the sufferer could inhale their fumes.[1]

The word *asthma* is derived from the Greek word *azein* meaning "to breathe hard."[2] Greek and Roman physicians managed individuals with gasping disorders with tailored treatment plans designs to balance the individuals' four "humors": yellow bile, black bile, blood, and phlegm. Today, we do not use the humoral theory of medicine, but we do recommend tailoring the patient's asthma plan to his or her unique situation.

It could be argued that our understanding of the condition had not advanced tremendously from ancient times until Hyde Salter, a London physician, described asthma as "paroxysmal dyspnoea of a peculiar character, generally periodic with intervals of healthy respiration between the attacks," in his *Treatise on Asthma: Its Pathology and Treatment*, published in 1860.[3] Salter, like many practitioners well into the 1980s, viewed asthma as an intermittent, acute condition.

It didn't help matters that Sir William Osler called asthma a "neurotic affection" in 1892.[4] Osler did, however, identify airway dysfunction and pathological changes in the lung such as bronchial mucosal edema, inflammation, and the production of gelatinous mucus as symptoms of the condition. He also noted that exposure to a "bizarre and extraordinary variety of circumstances" including airway infections and animal exposures induced the paroxysm. Many of the clinical descriptors Osler assigned to asthma we still use today, including spasms of the bronchial muscles, swelling of the bronchial mucosal membrane, inflammation of the smaller airway, and hay fever, which has many resemblances to asthma. He also noted that the affectation runs in families and he correctly identified that the illness often begins in childhood and sometimes lasts into old age.

What has changed in recent years is that we no longer think of asthma as a collection of intermittent symptoms, but as a chronic syndrome. This shift in our point of reference has changed the way we treat the disease. The idea of controlling asthma and preventing acute exacerbations has taken center stage and is the focus of today's treatment regimens.[5]

The Global Impact of Asthma

The Global Initiative for Asthma (GINA) estimates that nearly 300 million people worldwide have asthma.[6] Sharp increases in the occurrence of asthma in South Africa and the countries of the former Eastern Europe, including the Baltic States, particularly in children and the elderly have been noted in the last 10 years. This data however may be misleading; standardized data are still missing for many other countries in Africa, Asia, and South America, and data from some western countries may not be up to date. There are also data that suggest as countries become more westernized their asthma rates are increasing, leading investigators to hypothesize that asthma prevalence may increase globally to include an additional 100 million persons diagnosed with the illness by 2025.[7]

GINA defines the developing regions of the world as Africa, Central and South America, Asia, and the Pacific Basin. Asthma prevalence rates in these regions continue to rise significantly. Their investigators estimate that more than 40 million individuals in South and Central America have asthma. High prevalence rates have been reported in Peru (13.0%), Costa Rica (11.9%), Brazil (11.4%), and Ecuador (8.2%). In Africa, more than 50 million individuals are believed to have asthma. The highest asthma prevalence rates on this continent are found in South Africa (8.1%).

Almost 44 million people in the East Asia/Pacific region have asthma, although the prevalence rates, as well as reporting, vary markedly throughout the area. In China, a tenfold variation in the reported regional prevalence of asthma has been observed. Experts believe that significant increases in prevalence will be reported in China. This is attributed to China's population and the rate of economic development with associated lifestyle changes. They suggest that an absolute 2% increase in the prevalence of asthmatics in China would result in an additional 20 million asthmatics worldwide.

Surprisingly, the highest asthma rates worldwide are found in the United Kingdom and its former colonies. On average more than 1 in 15 individuals in the United Kingdom have asthma. An estimated 20,000 first or new episodes of asthma present each week to general practitioners in the United Kingdom.[8] Asthma is one of the leading causes of hospital admission in children with more than 75,000 emergency hospital admissions reported annually. The data shows that an estimated one in four people have severe or moderately severe asthma that might be relieved if treatment were reviewed and made more appropriate. One in 10 people living with severe or moderately severe asthma have inadequately controlled disease despite some of the best clinical and preventive management systems.

In North America, asthma statistics are also alarming. The prevalence of asthma symptoms and diagnosed asthma in Canada and the United States is among the highest in the world. One person in 10 in North America has asthma. Rates are higher in certain racial groups including African Americans and Hispanics compared with Caucasian children. Variances in urban compared with rural areas are also noted. If Canada and Mexico are removed from the statistics, the Centers for Disease Control and Prevention (CDC) in Atlanta, Georgia, report that in 2008 approximately 38.4 million people (10.2 million children and 28.2 million adults) in the United States had been diagnosed with asthma at some point during their lifetime. Of these, approximately 23.4 million individuals currently have asthma. In 2008, more than 4 million children within the United States (age 0–17 years) reported experiencing an asthma episode or attack during the previous 12 months (see Table 1.1).

Gender specific variances in asthma prevalence have been noted and seem to be age related. Overall, asthma is more common in females (13.5%) than in males (12.2%).[9] When specific calculations are made for age, male children (16%) were more likely than girls (11%) to have ever been diagnosed with asthma.[10]

Racial differences in the prevalence of asthma have also been documented. African American children report a 21.1% asthma rate compared to a 13.0% rate for Caucasian children in the United States. In adults, the numbers are a little more comparable with African Americans reporting 13.6% compared to Caucasians at 12.9% (see Table 1.2).

TABLE 1.1 Lifetime Asthma Population Estimates in Thousands by Age, United States: National Health Interview Survey, 2008

				Age (years)							
						15–34					
Characteristic†	*All Ages Total*	*Children Age < 18*	*Adults Age 18+*	*0–4*	*5–14*	*15–34*	*15–19*	*20–24*	*25–34*	*35–64*	*65+*
Total:	38,430	10,190	28,240	1,499	6,576	12,382	3,645	3,621	5,116	13,891	4,083
Male	17,867	6,184	11,683	1,031	3,919	6,082	2,038	1,733	2,312	5,271	1,564
Female	20,563	4,006	16,557	468	2,657	6,300	1,607	1,889	2,804	8,620	2,519
White Non-Hispanic:	25,308	5,356	19,952	676	3,347	8,171	2,449	2,387	3,334	9,961	3,153
Male	11,729	3,327	8,402	476	2,116	3,965	1,296	1,194	1,474	3,939	1,233
Female	13,579	2,029	11,550	200	1,231	4,206	1,153	1,193	1,860	6,022	1,920
Black Non-Hispanic:	5,819	2,283	3,536	325	1,587	1,757	497	523	737	1,763	387
Male	2,795	1,378	1,417	248	888	915	333	274	308	619	126
Female	3,024	905	2,119	77*	699	842	164	249	429	1,144	261
Other Non-Hispanic:	2,626	826	1,800	133*	554	774	210	206*	358	924	240
Male	1,279	543	735	102*	344	416	142*	104*	170*	321	95
Female	1,348	283	1,065	31*	210*	358	68*	**	188	603	145
Hispanic:	4,677	1,725	2,952	364	1,087	1,680	489	505	686	1,243	303
Male	2,065	937	1,128	205	571	786	266	160*	360	392	110*
Female	2,612	788	1,824	159*	516	894	222	345	327	851	192
Puerto Rican:[a]	943	344	598	44*	258	256	66*	76*	114	316	69*
Male	453	216	237	22*	176	109*	**	**	37*	104*	**
Female	490	128	361	**	82*	147	42*	**	77	211	27*

Mexican/Mexican-American:[a]	2,590	1,044	1,545	245	633	988	304	345	340	604	120
Male	1,042	490	553	118	272	444	177*	102*	165*	185	**
Female	1,547	555	993	127*	361	544	126*	243*	175	419	96
Region:											
Northeast	6,738	1,861	4,877	194	1,185	2,129	832	379	918	2,530	700
Midwest	9,725	2,509	7,216	427	1,596	3,189	851	1,094	1,244	3,567	945
South	12,885	3,798	9,087	614	2,456	3,962	1,164	1,175	1,623	4,486	1,367
West	9,081	2,022	7,059	264	1,338	3,101	798	974	1,330	3,308	1,070
Ratio of Family Income to Poverty Threshold:											
0–.99	6,518	2,314	4,204	489	1,487	2,098	577	808	713	2,057	388
1.00–2.49	10,971	3,354	7,617	412	2,312	3,547	1,059	1,089	1,399	3,123	1,578
2.50–4.49	10,365	2,418	7,947	337	1,484	3,528	1,065	1,012	1,452	3,750	1,266
4.50 and above	10,576	2,103	8,473	261	1,293	3,210	945	713	1,552	4,962	851

All relative standard errors are < 30% unless otherwise indicated.

* Relative standard error of the estimate is 30%–50%; the estimate is unreliable.

** Relative standard error of the estimate exceeds 50%.

† Numbers within selected characteristics may not sum to total due to rounding.

[a] As a subset of Hispanic.

Source: National Health Interview Survey, National Center for Health Statistics, CDC, Compiled 1/25/2008. Available: http://www.cdc.gov/asthma/nhis/08/table1-1.htm. Accessed April 16, 2010.

TABLE 1.2 Lifetime Asthma Prevalence Percents by Age, United States: National Health Interview Survey, 2008

				Age (years)							
						15–34					
Characteristic	*All ages Total*	*Children Age < 18*	*Adults Age 18+*	*0–4*	*5–14*	*15–34*	*15–19*	*20–24*	*25–34*	*35–64*	*65+*
Total:	12.9	13.8	12.5	7.2	16.4	15.1	17.4	17.5	12.7	11.7	11.0
Male	12.2	16.4	10.7	9.8	19.0	14.8	19.4	16.6	11.5	9.1	9.8
Female	13.5	11.1	14.2	4.6	13.6	15.5	15.4	18.4	14.0	14.2	11.9
White Non-Hispanic:	12.9	13.0	12.9	6.1	14.8	16.7	19.4	18.7	14.1	12.0	10.6
Male	12.3	15.9	11.2	8.4	18.4	16.1	20.4	18.3	12.5	9.6	9.5
Female	13.6	10.0	14.5	3.7	11.1	17.2	18.3	19.2	15.7	14.3	11.4
Black Non-Hispanic:	15.8	21.1	13.6	11.1	26.4	15.8	16.6	18.1	14.0	13.0	12.4
Male	16.3	24.7	12.2	16.4	28.4	17.4	21.8	21.3	12.6	10.2	10.3
Female	15.4	17.3	14.7	5.4*	24.2	14.3	11.2	15.5	15.3	15.2	13.6
Other Non-Hispanic:	13.1	14.0	12.8	8.0*	17.4	12.7	14.3	14.1*	11.4	12.6	14.0
Male	13.2	17.8	11.1	12.7*	20.2	14.4	18.9	15.3*	11.7	9.1	12.5
Female	13.1	9.9	14.3	3.6*	14.1	11.3	9.5*	**	11.2	15.8	15.2
Hispanic:	10.1	10.9	9.7	7.2	13.0	10.8	12.7	14.0	8.4	8.4	11.7
Male	8.7	11.6	7.2	7.9	13.3	9.5	14.1	8.2	8.1	5.2	10.0*
Female	11.6	10.2	12.3	6.5*	12.6	12.2	11.4	20.9	8.8	11.8	13.0
Puerto Rican:[a]	21.1	22.7	20.3	10.5*	29.4	19.3	16.4	25.4*	18.3	20.5	22.6
Male	21.0	26.5	17.6	9.1*	37.2	19.7*	17.6*	28.7*	14.8*	14.3*	25.6*
Female	21.2	18.2	22.5	**	20.2*	19.1	15.7*	**	20.7	26.1	19.2*

Mexican/Mexican-American:[a]	8.7	9.7	8.1	7.0	11.2	9.4	11.4	14.4	6.2	6.9	8.5
Male	6.8	9.0	5.6	6.5	9.7	7.8	13.1*	7.9*	5.4*	4.1	**
Female	10.7	10.4	10.9	7.5*	12.7	11.2	9.6	21.9	7.2	9.9	11.5
Region:											
Northeast	13.3	15.2	12.7	6.0	17.9	16.8	23.4	11.5	15.8	12.0	9.9
Midwest	13.5	14.0	13.3	8.7	15.9	15.9	17.0	21.6	12.4	12.7	10.8
South	12.0	14.7	11.2	8.5	17.3	13.3	15.2	15.8	11.1	10.5	10.1
West	13.2	11.4	13.8	4.9	14.3	16.0	17.0	19.9	13.6	12.2	13.8
Ratio of Family Income to Poverty Threshold:[b]											
0–.99	16.4	17.0	16.0	10.7	21.0	14.9	14.4	17.2	13.2	18.8	12.2
1.00–2.49	13.1	13.9	12.8	6.1	17.2	14.6	17.1	16.9	12.1	12.2	11.6
2.50–4.49	12.6	12.6	12.5	6.5	13.9	15.9	20.3	18.6	12.6	11.2	11.5
4.50 and above	11.4	12.6	11.1	6.2	14.4	15.1	17.1	17.3	13.3	10.1	9.1

All relative standard errors are < 30% unless otherwise indicated.

* Relative standard error of the estimate is 30%–50%; the estimate is unreliable.

** Relative standard error of the estimate exceeds 50%.

[a] As a subset of Hispanic.

[b] Missing responses imputed.

Source: National Health Interview Survey, National Center for Health Statistics, CDC. Compiled 1/25/2008. Available: http://www.cdc.gov/asthma/nhis/08/table2-1.htm. Accessed April 16, 2010.

In 2008, 4.7 million Hispanic Americans reported having been diagnosed with asthma at some point in their lifetime.[11] Overall, Hispanic adults had lower rates of asthma than non-Hispanic white adults and non-Hispanic black adults. However, the data show significant variances among Hispanic subgroups. Specifically, Puerto Ricans reported an asthma rate of 21.1%, while Mexican/Mexican-Americans reported a rate of 8.7%.

Regionally, Americans in the Midwest report higher asthma rates (13.5%) compared to those in the Northeast (13.3%); the west (13.2%) and southern United States (12.0%) report even lower rates.

Socioeconomically, asthma is more often reported among persons with a family income in the lowest poverty levels. It has been hypothesized that families living at or below the poverty threshold are more likely to live in substandard housing and have higher exposure rates to pest-related allergen and asthma triggers.[12]

Hospitalization Rates

Trends show a growing number of hospitalizations that can be directly attributed to asthma, particularly for children. In Europe, acute asthma is the most common cause of hospital admissions among children.[13] The *Asthma in America* survey,[14] conducted by telephone from May 21 to July 7, 1998, identified that approximately 9% of asthma patients required hospitalization, 23% needed emergency department treatment, and 29% had to have an unscheduled emergency appointment because of their asthma. Hospitalization rates for African Americans are 50% higher than for Caucasian patients. In children the hospitalization rate can be 150% higher for African Americans than for Caucasians.[15] The data also shows that more women than men are hospitalized for asthma. An analysis of hospital discharge data from 2005 showed that 296,000 hospital discharges were reported for females, while 192,000 were reported for males.[16] The hospitalization discharge data from 1995–2005 also shows variations on age groups for asthma. For individuals younger than 15 years of age and those aged 15–44 years, hospital discharge rates declined. The rates for individuals 45–64 years of age have remained stable, while discharge rates for those 65 years of age and older have risen 33%.[9]

In 2005, a reported 12.8 million physician office visits, 1.3 million outpatient department visits, and almost 1.8 million emergency room visits were reported for or attributed to asthma; 1.1 million of the emergency room visits were for adults and 696,900 visits were for children.[9]

Mortality

Internationally, 180,000 deaths are attributable to asthma each year.[17] Although variations in asthma reporting somewhat skew this data, the World

Health Organization (WHO) reports that most asthma-related deaths occur in low- and lower- to middle-income countries. Worldwide asthma mortality rates have declined since the 1980s[8] (see Table 1.3).

In the United States, 3816 people died of asthma in 2004 and an estimated 3857 died in 2005.[18] Age-related variances were noted in the data, with individuals over the age of 65 being more likely to die from asthma than those in other age groups. Women were also more likely to succumb to their symptoms, with some 64% of asthma deaths in 2004 occurring in females. African Americans were more than three times more likely to die from asthma than Caucasians. Overall, however, there is some positive data as asthma deaths in the United States have been continuously declining for the past 6 years.[15]

What Does Asthma Cost?

The economic implications of a diagnosis of asthma are staggering. The WHO has reported the annual costs of asthma exceed those of tuberculosis and HIV combined.[16,19] These costs are usually attributed to poor asthma control and disease management, with a disproportionate number of patients using

TABLE 1.3 Highest Documented Asthma Mortality Rates in the World*

Ranking	*Country*	*Proportion of Population (%)*
1.	China	36.7
2.	Russia	28.6
3.	Uzbekistan	27.2
4.	Albania	20.8
5.	South Africa	18.5
6.	Singapore	16.1
7.	Romania	14.7
8.	Mexico	14.5
9.	Malta	11.6
10.	Colombia	10.1

Note: The United States ranks 25th on this listing with a rate of 5.2 case fatalities per 100,000 asthmatics.

* The asthma mortality comparisons between the different countries has been made using mortality rates in the 5–34-year age group. The authors used the WHO country-specific mortality data for ICD codes 490 to 493 and data from the two most recent years in which it was available for each country.

Adapted from: Masoli M, Fabian D, Holt S, et al. Global Initiative for Asthma (GINA) program: the global burden, 2004. Available at: http://www.ginasthma.com.

a larger portion of the healthcare dollars.[20,21] The evaluation of asthma costs considers both direct costs, which include the cost of medications and treatment, and indirect costs, such as loss of school or work days and decrease in productivity. In Europe the estimated total cost of asthma is $21.65 billion per year. Outpatient costs account for approximately $4.65 billion of these expenses, while medications account for $4.4 billion annually. Indirect costs of $11.99 billion are directly attributed to poor asthma control. In England, for example, 69% of parents or partners of parents of children with asthma report taking time off from work because of their child's asthma-related complications. Thirteen percent report that they have lost a job because of their child's asthma.[22]

In the United States the annual economic cost of asthma is $19.7 billion ($14.7 billion in direct healthcare costs and $5 billion for indirect costs). The *Asthma in America* survey provides a snapshot of the indirect costs of asthma in the United States. The survey interviewed 2509 adults with asthma or parents of children with asthma, as well as more than 700 healthcare providers from across America. The survey found that when compared to the general public, the people with asthma averaged 75% more sick day usage. The respondents who reported having severe asthma were shown to have spent approximately 4 days in bed in the previous month due to their asthma. Almost half of the adults with asthma (47%) said that their disease has caused them to change their expectations about what they are able to do, with almost two-thirds (64%) of respondents admitting that their health limits their activities. In the general public only 1 in 4 (26%) people believe their health limits their activities. The true impact of asthma on an individual's daily routine, also known as their activities of daily living, is hard to quantify. On days when their asthma is less active, there may be minimal impact on the individual's behavior. On more active asthma days, basic activities such as walking to the restroom and eating may be difficult. The asthmatics surveyed noted that their asthma caused limitations in sports and recreation (48%), normal physical exertion (36%), sleeping (36%), and general lifestyle overall (31%). Nearly half of the asthmatics surveyed (45%) said there are things that they would like to do that they cannot do because of their asthma.[23]

A partner study, *Children and Asthma in America,* conducted by telephone interview from February to May 2004, collected data from 801 children (or their care providers), 4–18 years of age with a current asthma diagnosis. This data shows that for many children their asthma is uncontrolled. In the month prior to the survey, 67%, or about two-thirds, of the children had experienced daytime, nighttime, or exercise-induced symptoms; 19%, or 1 in 5 children, had experienced daytime symptoms three times a week to daily; and 22% reported nighttime symptoms once a week to daily. More than half of the children (54%) had missed school or daycare in the past year because of their asthma with an average of nearly 4 days missed. This had a negative impact on the parents as well, with 39% reporting that they had missed work in the past year due to their child's asthma. Poorly controlled asthma was shown to have a direct negative impact on the quality of the children's lives. When surveyed, 62% of the children reported that they were limited by their asthma and in their activities of daily living as well as participating in sports, having pets, sleeping, attending school, and/or joining in outdoor activities with friends and family.[22]

Managing Asthma

As is apparent from this data, the burden of asthma on those with the condition as well as the healthcare systems and economies of the world is huge. Differences in healthcare systems, standards of living, and access to care prevent any easy global fix for the problem. Asthma is also not a healthcare priority for many nations, though significant proportions of their populations suffer from the illness. In Africa for example, most governments concentrate their healthcare efforts on reversing poor nutrition, poor housing, and halting the spread of infectious diseases such as HIV/AIDS. Many governments lack the resources to tackle these priorities, let alone asthma.[8]

GINA guidelines, updated in December 2009, stress the importance of implementing guidelines at the national and local level that include a wide variety of professional groups and other stakeholders, establishing a system of care that evaluates the effectiveness and quality of care delivered, and focusing on the most cost-effective management approaches that are available to as many patients as possible.[23] These guidelines include a detailed implementation plan as well as a checklist on the issues for national and local asthma implementation strategies to assist the healthcare systems.[24]

In the United States, there are several options available for improving asthma control (see Box 1.1). Healthy People 2010, a national initiative to improve overall health, identified asthma as a significant respiratory illness and has established goals for better management of the disease. The program advises that the effective management of asthma includes four components: avoiding or controlling the factors/triggers that may make asthma worse, utilizing appropriate medications tailored to the severity of the disease, effective and objective monitoring of the disease by the patient and the healthcare professional, and patient-focused disease management.[25]

America Breathing Easier is part of the CDC's National Asthma Control Program based on the Healthy People 2010 goals for asthma.[9] This program funds state, city, and school programs to improve asthma awareness; creates, establishes, and expands surveillance systems, trains health professionals, and educates individuals with asthma and their families and community.

The American Lung Association has several patient and professional tools to assist in asthma management, as well as active state and regional chapters that provide direct support at the local level.

Box 1.1 Useful Asthma Resources

The Global Initiative for Asthma (GINA)
http://www.ginasthma.com/

American Lung Association
http://www.lungusa.org/

Centers for Disease Control and Prevention: Asthma
http://www.cdc.gov/asthma/

National Asthma Education and Prevention Program (United States)
http://www.nhlbi.nih.gov/about/naepp/

Guidelines for the Diagnosis and Management of Asthma (EPR 3; United States)
http://www.nhlbi.nih.gov/guidelines/asthma/

NHLBI: Physician Asthma Care Education
http://www.nhlbi.nih.gov/health/prof/lung/asthma/pace/

American Academy of Allergy, Asthma, and Immunology
http://www.aaaai.org/

American College of Allergy, Asthma, and Immunology
http://www.acaai.org/

American Association for Respiratory Care
http://www.aarc.org/

American College of Chest Physicians
http://www.chestnet.org/

American Thoracic Society
http://www.thoracic.org/

Association of Asthma Educators
http://www.asthmaeducators.org/

Practitioners in the United States can also turn to the National Heart, Lung, and Blood Institute (NHLBI). A division of the National Institutes of Health (NIH) the NHLBI manages several initiatives that can assist asthma patients and their care providers. Among these is the National Asthma Education and Prevention Program (NAEPP). This agency has established goals of raising asthma awareness as a serious chronic disease; as well as insuring effective diagnosis and treatment. Administered and coordinated by the NHLBI, the NAEPP works with intermediaries such as major medical associations, voluntary health organizations, and community programs to educate patients, health professionals, and the general public. The NHLBI is also the organization that convenes the "Expert Panel" that develops the guidelines for asthma used in the United States. The most current version of the Expert Panel Report is Version 3 (EPR-3). The Physician Asthma Care Education (PACE) program, also supported by the NHLBI, is a two-part interactive, multimedia educational seminar. The goal of this program is to improve physician awareness, ability, and use of communication and therapeutic techniques to reduce the effects of asthma on children and their families. PACE provides instruction on how to document, code, and improve asthma counseling reimbursement for providers as well. The program can be conducted at the local level and involves two 2.5-hour interactive sessions, which should be held one week apart.

Many state and local health departments, as well as school systems, have developed programs to increase asthma awareness and improve care. Practitioners are encouraged to contact their local agencies to determine their available resources.

References

1. National Library of Medicine. Origins of Western Medicine. http://www.nlm.nih.gov/hmd/breath/breath_exhibit/MindBodySpirit/origins.html. Accessed April 6, 2009.
2. Soukhanov A, ed. *Encarta World English Dictionary*. New York: St. Martin's Press; 1999. http://encarta.msn.com/encnet/features/dictionary/dictionaryhome.aspx. Accessed April 6, 2009.
3. Salter HH. *On Asthma: Its Pathology and Treatment*. London: John Churchill; 1860.
4. Osler W. *Principles and Practice of Medicine*. New York: D. Appleton and Co.; 1892.
5. National Heart, Lung, and Blood Institute. *National Asthma Education and Prevention Program Expert Panel Report 3: Guidelines for the Diagnosis and Management of Asthma Full Report 2007*. http://www.nhlbi.nih.gov/guidelines/asthma/asthsumm.pdf. Accessed April 2, 2009.
6. The Global Initiative for Asthma. *2008 Update of the GINA Report*. Global Strategy for Asthma Management and Prevention. http://www.ginasthma.com/. Accessed April 6, 2009.
7. Masoli M, Fabian D, Holt S, et al. Global Initiative for Asthma (GINA) program: the global burden of asthma: executive summary of the GINA Dissemination Committee report. *Allergy*. 2004;59:469–478.
8. Masoli M, Fabian D, Holt S, et al. Global Initiative for Asthma (GINA) program: the global burden 2004. http://www.ginasthma.com. Accessed April 9, 2009.
9. Centers for Disease Control and Prevention's National Asthma Control Program. America Breathing Easier. http://www.cdc.gov/asthma/NACP.htm. Accessed April 15, 2009.
10. US Department of Health and Human Services, Centers for Disease Control and Prevention Vital and Health Statistics. Summary Health Statistics for U.S. Children: National Health Interview Survey, 2008. Series 10, No 244. December

2009. Available: http://www.cdc.gov/nchs/data/series/sr_10/sr10_242.pdf. Accessed April 13, 2010.

11. Centers for Disease Control and Prevention. Trends in Asthma Morbidity and Mortality. *National Center for Health Statistics, National Health Interview Survey Raw Data, 1997–2006*. Analysis performed by American Lung Association Research and Program Services using SPSS and SUDAAN software. http://www.lungusa.org/atf/cf/%7B7A8D42C2-FCCA-4604-8ADE-7F5D5E762256%7D/ASTHMA1.PDF. Accessed April 1, 2009.
12. Cohn RD, Arbes SJ Jr, Jaramillo R, Reid LH, Zeldin DC. National prevalence and exposure risk for cockroach allergen in U.S. households. *Environ Health Perspect*. 2006;114(4):522–6.
13. European Lung Foundation. *European Lung White Book*. Brussels, Belgium: European Respiratory Society and the European Lung Foundation; 2003.
14. *Asthma in America: A Landmark Survey*. GlaxoSmithKline; 1998. http://www.asthmainamerica.com. Accessed April 6, 2009.
15. Beasley R. The burden of asthma with specific reference to the United States. *J Allergy Clin Immunol*. 2002;109(5):S482–S489.
16. American Lung Association. *Trends in Asthma Morbidity and Mortality*. November 2007. http://www.lungusa.org/atf/cf/%7B7A8D42C2-FCCA-4604-8ADE-7F5D5E762256%7D/ASTHMA1.PDF. Accessed April 1, 2009.
17. World Health Organization. WHO fact sheet 206: bronchial asthma. http://www.who.int/mediacentre/factsheets/fs206/en. Accessed April 6, 2009.
18. Centers for Disease Control and Prevention. National Center for Health Statistics. National Vital Statistics Reports. Deaths: Final Data for 2004. August 21, 2007;55(19). http://www.cdc.gov/nchs/products/pubs/pubd/hestats/asthma03-05/asthma03-05.htm. Accessed on April 14, 2009.
19. Braman SS. The Global Burden of Asthma. *Chest*. 2006;130(1):4S–12S.
20. Sennhauser FH, Braun-Fahrländer C, Wildhaber JH. The burden of asthma in children: a European perspective. *Paediatr Respir Rev*. 2005;6(1):2–7.
21. Marcus P, Arnold RJ, Ekins S, et al. A retrospective randomized study of asthma control in the US: results of the CHARIOT study. *Curr Med Res Opin*. 2008;24(12):3443–52.
22. *Children and Asthma in America: A Landmark Survey*. GlaxoSmithKline; 2004. http://www.asthmainamerica.com. Accessed April 6, 2009.
23. The Global Initiative for Asthma (GINA). *Global strategy for asthma management and prevention*. Updated 2009. http://www.ginasthma.com. Accessed April 9, 2010.
24. The Global Initiative for Asthma (GINA). *Global strategy for asthma management and prevention*. Updated 2008. http://www.ginasthma.com. Accessed April 9, 2009.
25. US Department of Health and Human Services. Respiratory Diseases. In: *Healthy People 2010*. http://www.healthypeople.gov/Document/HTML/Volume2/24Respiratory.htm#_Toc489704825. Accessed April 15, 2009.

2

Defining Asthma

LEARNING OBJECTIVES

- Discuss the definition and clinical characteristics of asthma
- Review the signs and symptoms of asthma
- Identify the different types of asthma
- Review the association between allergies and asthma
- Identify common asthma triggers
- Review methods to control asthma triggers

KEY WORDS

airflow obstruction
bronchial hyperresponsiveness
airway inflammation
work-related asthma (WRA)
occupational asthma (OA)
trigger
atopy
allergen
intercostal retractions
gastroesophageal reflux disease (GERD)
obstructive sleep apnea (OSA)
aspirin-exacerbated respiratory disease (AERD)
exercise-induced bronchospasm
antigen
allergic cascade
immunoglobulin (Ig)
mast cells/basophils
leukotriene
dander
hygiene hypothesis
high-efficiency particulate air (HEPA) filter

What Is Asthma?

Asthma is usually thought of as a disease characterized by intermittent wheezing in response to an irritant or allergen. Unfortunately, many asthmatics also think of the condition in this way. This mindset has led to treatment of symptoms of asthma as they occur and does not address the underlying causes of the condition. Appropriate treatment of the underlying causes of asthma can prevent the symptoms from occurring and significantly improve the individual's quality of life. There are numerous examples of asthmatics who participate in professional sports or who have successful careers because their asthma is "controlled" and does not impact their daily activities.

Physiologically asthma is a complex cascade of conditions and interactions that lead to acute airflow obstruction, increased mucous production, bronchial hyperresponsiveness, and airway inflammation.[1] Each of these interactions and their manifestations can be slightly different depending on the individual and can even vary in severity in the same individual due to their internal physiologic environment and external factors. It is these physiologic interactions that result in the wheezing and breathing difficulties that the individual experiences and we call asthma.

The clinical characteristics of asthma are defined as the occurrence of symptoms and the presence of airway obstruction, inflammation, and hyperresponsiveness.[2]

Signs and Symptoms

Defining the signs and symptoms of asthma is challenging as the manifestations from a clinical perspective vary from person to person (see Table 2.1). While most asthma patients present with wheezing, some do not. As clinicians, we often also use the terms exacerbation or episode to define an "attack" of wheezing or shortness of breath in an asthmatic.

Different Types of Asthma

Childhood Asthma

Asthma is the most common chronic disorder in children and, if untreated, has a direct negative impact on the quality of the child's life. While most children with asthma present with the traditional symptom of wheezing, many do not. A persistent cough is a common asthmatic symptom that is often overlooked in children. A child who coughs during or after vigorous playing, running, or crying may have asthma. Recurrent coughing at night is also a common sign seen in asthmatic children. Many of these children will also report having difficulty sleeping and may have difficulty staying awake during the day or concentrating on their school work.[3,4]

TABLE 2.1 Asthma Symptoms and Severity

Common Asthma Symptoms	*Symptoms That May Be Associated with Asthma*	*Symptoms of Severe Asthma*
Peak flow numbers in the caution/yellow range (usually 50%–80% of personal best) Cough with or without mucous production; often worse at night or early in the morning, making it hard to sleep	Abnormal breathing pattern characterized by prolonged expiration	Peak flow numbers in the danger/red zone (usually < 50% of personal best) Cyanosis
Shortness of breath that gets worse with exercise or activity	Breathing temporarily stops Posturing (hunched shoulders)	Alterations in consciousness (i.e., drowsiness, confusion) during an asthma exacerbation
Intercostal retractions	Chest pain	Extreme difficulty breathing
Wheezing • Usually begins suddenly • Episodic in nature • May go away on its own • May be worse at night or in early morning • Gets worse when breathing in cold air • Gets worse with exercise • Gets worse with heartburn (reflux) • Improves when using appropriate medications	Nasal flaring Tightness in the chest	Tachycardia Severe anxiety due to shortness of breath Sweating

Adapted from: National Library of Medicine. Medline Plus: Asthma. http://www.nlm.nih.gov/medlineplus/ency/article/000141.htm. Accessed April 24, 2009.

National Jewish Health. Asthma: Signs and Symptoms. http://www.nationaljewish.org/healthinfo/conditions/asthma/symptoms.aspx. Accessed April 24, 2009.

A young child may say that their chest feels funny, or that their chest hurts when they run and play. They may be especially irritable and cough. These may be signs of asthma and should be evaluated if they are recurrent. Detecting asthma in infants is also difficult. Babies cannot respond to our questions, and there are no definitive testing procedures for infants. If the baby grunts, snorts, or has difficulty breathing while feeding, he or she may be experiencing airway inflammation and/or obstruction. Any child or infant who experiences frequent coughing or respiratory infections should be evaluated for asthma.[5]

Hidden asthma is a term applied to children who have subclinical asthma that is often difficult to detect by assessing the usual signs and symptoms. Children with breathing difficulties and/or recurrent coughing, who self-limit their physical activities, should be assessed for airway obstruction and underlying hidden asthma.[6]

One of the most common questions asked about childhood asthma is "Can you outgrow it?" The answer is: maybe. Results of studies to date have been mixed. In one study researchers identified that 85% of infants hospitalized for wheezing did seem to outgrow their symptoms by adolescence. However some 30%–40% of these individuals had asthma reemerge as young adults.[7] These findings, suggesting that childhood asthma is a predictor for asthma in early adulthood, have been confirmed by other studies as well.[8] Several factors that may help predict if the asthma may remerge have been also identified.[9] Sensitization to house dust mites, airway hyperresponsiveness, female gender, smoking, and early age of initial onset of asthma, may predict asthma persistence or relapse of symptoms later in life.[8,9]

There are studies that suggest that even though individuals have "outgrown" their asthma (i.e., they no longer have exacerbations) they continue to have changes in their airway structure and abnormal pulmonary function testing when measured in adulthood. Whether these findings are "hold-overs" from their childhood asthma or ongoing subclinical progression is unclear.[10]

Can You Outgrow Asthma?

Some children continue to have asthma throughout their life; others have improvements in their asthma symptoms during adolescence and young adulthood, and their asthma does not return; still others improve in adolescence only to have their symptoms return in midlife or later.[11]

Work-Related/Occupational Asthma

Work-related asthma (WRA) is defined as an asthmatic airway response to dust, vapors, gases, or fumes that exist or are encountered in the workplace. This condition can be further subdivided into work-exacerbated asthma (WEA), which is aggravation of preexisting asthma or occupational asthma (OA)—asthma that is directly caused by a workplace exposure. To further complicate matters, OA is further defined in a variety of ways. Most medical texts differentiate between sensitizer-induced asthma and irritant-induced asthma.[12] Sensitizer-induced asthma refers to individuals who have reversible airflow limitation caused by sensitization to a substance encountered at work that involves a latent period (this can be called immunologic asthma as well). Put another way, the individual develops asthma over a period of time in response to exposure to an irritant. More than 250 agents have been documented as causing immunologic occupational asthma.[13] These agents are divided into high-molecular-weight (HMW) compounds (> 5000 Da) and low-molecular-weight (LMW) compounds (< 5000 Da). The HMW compounds act as complete antigens in and of themselves, whereas the LMW compounds react with proteins (autologous or heterologous) to form a complete antigen. Data has shown that OA may account for 25% or more of first time asthma diagnosis in adults.[14]

The term *irritant-induced asthma* is used to describe individuals who develop persistent asthma symptoms and nonspecific airway hyperresponsiveness after a single short-term, high-intensity inhalational exposure. Irritant-induced asthma is also called reactive airways dysfunction syndrome (RADS).[15]

A nonimmunologic type of occupational asthma (without latency) has also been defined. This type of asthma refers to asthma that can occur in response to either single or multiple exposures to irritants at concentrations high enough to induce airway injury and inflammation.[16,17]

Organic dust-induced airways disease is yet another type of work-related pulmonary illness. This condition is related to occupational exposure to organic dusts such as cotton, flax, hemp, jute, sisal, and various grains. This family of diseases is not actually asthma. Individuals who develop these conditions are more likely to present with chronic bronchitis and chronic airflow limitation while lacking the presence of airway eosinophilia. Symptoms usually include wheezing, tightness in the chest, coughing, and/or shortness of breath.[18]

The diagnosis of WRA differs from the standard method of diagnosing asthma. In addition to assessing the individual's symptoms, a diagnosis of WRA requires an assessment of the individual's workplace and identification of the irritant when possible. Treatment of WRA does not differ from the treatment of other types of asthma. A stepwise approach based on the severity of individuals' asthma and their level of control is used. When possible, removal of the irritant and prevention of further exposure are recommended.

Nocturnal Asthma, Gastroesophageal Reflux Disease, and Obstructive Sleep Apnea

There is debate as to whether or not nocturnal asthma is a distinct type of asthma in and of itself. There is data that suggests that nighttime asthma symptoms are more an indication of poorly controlled asthma in general.[19] It is clear that nighttime awakenings in children with asthma may affect school attendance and performance, as well as work attendance by their parents.[19] The current U.S. guidelines include nocturnal asthma as one of the four key symptoms that should be assessed when reviewing a patient's history.[2]

The occurrence of nocturnal asthma symptoms has been associated with gastroesophageal reflux disease (GERD). Data has shown that GERD during sleep can contribute to nocturnal asthma.[20] Treatment of GERD with a proton pump inhibitor does not directly improve the asthma symptoms, improve pulmonary function results, or reduce the use of rescue medications. It does however reduce the number of asthma exacerbations and improve the quality of life for asthmatic patients.[21] Therefore, the current asthma treatment guidelines recommend the assessment for, and medical management of, GERD.

Obstructive sleep apnea (OSA) is another condition that has been associated with nocturnal asthma. Though OSA and nocturnal asthma are distinct entities, there is data that suggests they are linked. The indirect effect on dyspnea of OSA-induced cardiac dysfunction coupled with neuromechanical bronchoconstriction, gastroesophageal reflux, and inflammation may lead to worsening asthma control in patients with OSA. It has also been hypothesized that vascular endothelial growth factor-induced airway angiogenesis, leptin-related airway changes, and OSA-induced weight gain may also contribute to poor asthma control.[22] There is a growing body of evidence that suggests that continuous positive airway pressure (CPAP) to treat OSA has a positive impact on asthma control. The exact mechanisms, however, have yet to be defined.[23,24]

Exercise-Induced Bronchospasm

Exercise-induced bronchospasm (EIB) is a term that is used to describe acute, transient airway narrowing in response to exercise. There is debate as to whether EIB can be clearly defined as a type of asthma in and of itself or as a symptom of asthma in general. Some 50%–90% of all individuals with asthma have airways that are hyperreactive to exercise.[25] Yet there is also data that shows that 10% of individuals with EIB are not known to have any other type of asthma symptoms or have the tendency to develop allergic diseases or experience an allergic reaction. This tendency is known as atopy.[26]

We do know that EIB is most likely to occur during and after exercise and is defined as airway narrowing in response to exercise.[27] Left untreated EIB can cause individuals with asthma to limit their activities and the current guidelines recommend that asthmatic patients be assessed for EIB. Patients who present with EIB should also be followed regularly to ensure that they have no symptoms of asthma or reductions in their peak expiratory flow (PEF) at other times when they are not exercising.[2]

Diagnosing EIB can be challenging. Individuals will usually have a history of coughing, shortness of breath, chest pain or tightness, or endurance problems during exercise. They may or may not report wheezing. These findings are suggestive of a diagnosis of EIB. Diagnosis is usually made by an exercise challenge test. Findings of a 15% decrease in PEF or FEV_1 (with measurements taken before and after exercise at 5-minute intervals for 20–30 minutes) is compatible with a diagnosis of EIB.

Asthma During Pregnancy and Menses-Related Asthma

Asthma is not a contraindication for pregnancy. However, an expectant mother whose asthma is poorly controlled may face a higher risk for herself and her baby should she experience an exacerbation. Studies have shown that during pregnancy the severity of asthma often changes. The data is pretty evenly divided. For approximately one-third of women their asthma becomes worse during pregnancy; for one-third of asthmatic mothers to be, their asthma becomes less severe; and the remaining one-third report no changes in their asthma severity during pregnancy.[28–30] Poorly controlled asthma can have a serious impact on the baby, resulting in increased perinatal mortality, increased chance of premature birth, and low birth weight.[29,30] Pregnant women with asthma should be followed closely and adjustments made to their medications and asthma action plan to insure good control of their asthma and reduce the risks of adverse outcomes to the baby and the mother.[2,30]

Variations in asthma severity during menstruation and premenstrual exacerbations have also been documented in many women.[31] While this may suggest a hormonal component to these exacerbations, there is not enough data to confirm this relationship at this time. The term menses-related asthma has been applied to this form of asthma.

Treatment-Resistant Asthma

For most asthmatics corticosteroids are used to control their airway inflammation and mange their asthma. Treatment-resistant asthma is the term used to describe the 5%–10% of individuals who do not respond to corticosteroid therapy.[32] While the condition can be seen at any asthma severity level, it is most commonly found in cases of severe asthma.[33] It was initially believed that this treatment resistance was related to a defect in the individual's response to corticosteroids that restricts the anti-inflammatory effects of these medications. Studies have shown however that there are multiple components and mechanisms of steroid resistance. Abnormalities in histone deacetylation pathways, overexpression of the alternative, nonfunctional glucocorticoid receptor β, or transcription-factor interference with corticosteroid binding to the functional glucocorticoid receptor α have all been documented.[34] It has also been suggested that some treatment-resistant asthmatics have variations in the type of inflammation associated with their asthma that may account for the variations in corticosteroid response.[35]

Aspirin-Sensitive Asthma, Aspirin-Induced Asthma, and Aspirin-Exacerbated Respiratory Disease

It has been estimated that approximately 21% of adults and 5% of children who have asthma experience asthma exacerbations in response to aspirin and other nonsteroidal anti-inflammatory drugs (NSAIDs).[2,36] The condition has come to be known by several names including aspirin-sensitive asthma (ASA), aspirin-induced asthma (AIA), and aspirin-exacerbated respiratory disease (AERD). It is known that the prevalence of the condition increases as the patient ages and/or has a higher severity of asthma.[37] Because of the risk of Reye's syndrome, children and teenagers should not use aspirin or products containing aspirin-related medications for flu-like symptoms or chickenpox without first consulting their physician. Because ASA has been identified in a small number of children with asthma, parents should consult their physician before giving aspirin to their asthmatic child.

Many adult patients with ASA follow a similar pattern of disease development. They typically report rhinitis and profuse rhinorrhea, during their 30s and 40s. This evolves into chronic nasal congestion. Upon physical examination, many are found to have nasal polyps in addition to chronic hyperplastic eosinophilic sinusitis.[38] These findings are usually precursors of the early stages of onset for asthma and aspirin hypersensitivity. Aspirin hypersensitivity is defined as an acute, often severe, asthma episode, usually accompanied by rhinorrhea, nasal obstruction, conjunctival irritation, and scarlet flush of the head and neck that develops within minutes or within 1–2 hours following ingestion of aspirin. It is believed that any medication that acts as a cyclooxygenase-1 (COX-1) inhibitor can induce an asthmatic response; therefore, several NSAIDs that are COX-1 inhibitors can also cause ASA.

While the exact mechanism by which these medications trigger bronchoconstriction remains unknown, data has shown significant eosinophilic inflammation, epithelial disruption, increased cytokine production (particularly interleukin-5 [IL-5]), and upregulation of adhesion molecules occurring in the airways of patients with ASA.[39] Because many of these patients seem to have an underlying inflammatory disease of the entire respiratory tract, the term aspirin-exacerbated respiratory disease has also been developed to describe this condition.

Once an individual develops aspirin sensitivity, they should be advised to avoid aspirin and COX-1 inhibitors that could aggravate their condition. Should these individuals require an NSAID, a cyclooxygenase-2 (COX-2) inhibitor may be considered; however, physician supervision and observation for at least 1 hour after administration are advised.[40] Acetaminophen, salsalate, or the COX-2 inhibitor celecoxib are alternatives to aspirin that usually do not cause acute bronchoconstriction in aspirin-sensitive patients.

Practitioners should query adult asthmatic patients about their history of symptoms including bronchoconstriction following the use of aspirin and other NSAIDs. If they report having had a reaction to any of these medications, they should be informed of the potential for all of these drugs to precipitate severe and even fatal asthma exacerbations. In addition, adult patients who have severe persistent asthma or nasal polyps should be counseled regarding the potential risk of using these medications.[2] Utilization of an aspirin challenge test as a diagnostic tool for ASA is not recommended as it is associated with a high risk of potentially fatal consequences.[41] Aspirin desensitization therapy has been used as a treatment for ASA. The daily use of aspirin is believed to control inflammation, reduce upper-airway mucosal congestion, and delay or slow nasal polyp formation. If desensitization therapy is successful the individual is usually placed on a daily regimen of aspirin therapy.[42] It is believed that the desensitization can be maintained indefinitely as long as the individual takes the daily aspirin treatment.[43] Desensitization therapy should only be conducted by experienced practitioners with full resuscitation capabilities.

Vocal Cord Dysfunction

Vocal cord dysfunction (VCD) is characterized by paroxysmal adduction of the vocal cords, resulting in airway restriction and is often misdiagnosed as asthma. Individuals report stridor, shortness of breath, wheezing, cough, and exertional dyspnea in some cases.[44] These misdiagnosed asthmatics are often placed on an asthma action plan that does not control their symptoms. As their "asthma progresses," the medication levels in their asthma action plans are usually increased to no avail.[45] Vocal cord dysfunction is diagnosed by direct visualization of the vocal cord movement. Speech therapy is the treatment of choice for individuals with VCD.[46]

Trigger-Related Asthma

Trigger-related asthma is a term used to describe a family of asthmatic phenotypes that includes asthma that is "activated" or caused in response to a particular irritant or trigger. The term would encompass allergic asthma, occupational asthma, aspirin-induced asthma, pregnancy/menses-related asthma, and exercise-induced asthma.[33]

Allergic Asthma

Allergic asthma is perhaps the most common type of asthma. This variety of asthma can present at any age, though it usually begins in early childhood. A family history of asthma and early exposure to allergens are considered to be the most common etiologies of the condition. Essentially, allergic asthma is defined as asthmatic symptoms in response to an allergen irritant. Allergic asthma is generally associated with airway inflammation, though a clear definition of what constitutes allergic asthma has not been established. It has been suggested that a definition of allergic asthma should include demonstration of both specific IgE, in the form of a positive skin-prick test or radioallergosorbent test, and a history of allergic symptoms in response to a trigger.[33]

Atopic Asthma and Extrinsic Asthma

The terms atopic asthma and extrinsic asthma are often used interchangeably with allergic asthma. Specifically, the word atopy refers to an allergic hypersensitivity that can cause a reaction either in the pulmonary system as allergic asthma or in the skin as dermatitis. A more clinical definition is a genetic predisposition to the development of an IgE-mediated response to an allergen. Atopy is believed to be the most significant identifiable predisposing factor for the development of asthma.[2]

Allergens and Asthma

The association between allergies and asthma has been clearly documented.[47] When an allergen or infective agent enters the body via the respiratory system a series of reactions in the immune system known as the "allergic cascade" is triggered. The respiratory system and in particular the bronchi begin to recruit inflammatory cells from the bloodstream into the bronchial wall. These inflammatory cells secrete proteins that identify and bind to the allergen and/or potentially invading organism. Concurrently, swelling of the bronchial wall, and an increase in bronchial secretions and airway constriction can occur. The main components in the allergic cascade are immunoglobulin (Ig), also more commonly known as antibodies; and mast cells/basophils and chemical mediators. A more detailed explanation of airway inflammation and its components are discussed in Chapter 3.

Infections Versus Allergies: An Immunologic View

> The body's initial response to an infection is the same as that to an allergen. T lymphocytes race to the site of the invasion, determine what type of antigen they are dealing with, and then call for back up. The difference lies in the type of T-helper (i.e., Th1 or Th2) cell the T lymphocyte calls in for reinforcements. If the T lymphocyte determines that it is dealing with an allergen it calls in Th2 cells. If the T lymphocyte determines it is battling an infection, it calls in Th1 cells.[48]

Allergen Triggers

An allergen trigger is any substance that can initiate the atopic (IgE-mediated) response in the body. The most common triggers are mold, animal proteins (from skin or saliva), dust mites, cockroach particles, and pollen.

Some Common Triggers and How to Control Them

It is impractical to think that we can control an individual's exposure to potential asthma triggers 100% of the time. Steps can be taken, however, to minimize their exposure and to manage the impact of an allergen trigger. The first step in any successful allergen avoidance plan is to identify the allergen. This may not be as easy as it seems. A detailed history of the patient's past allergen/asthmatic responses coupled with any available clinical data will assist in clarifying the potential risks. Knowing the risks coupled with careful patient self-monitoring and a proactive asthma management plan can help achieve allergen-triggered asthma control. The current U.S. guidelines recommend an allergen-control education program, not only for patients but also for their immediate family.

High-Efficiency Particulate Air Filters, Electrostatic Precipitating Filters, and Air Duct Cleaning

High-efficiency particulate air (HEPA) filters can remove approximately 99.97% of airborne particles in the 0.3 micrometers (μm) diameter range. These devices operate by pulling air through the filter and trapping the particles in the filter material. The replacement filters can be expensive and should be changed regularly to prevent bacterial contamination. Electrostatic precipitating filters, sometimes also called plate precipitators, operate using a dual stage process. The first stage produces a charged particle that is emitted into the air and attracts particulate matter. The second stage pulls air over a series of collection plates that "catch" the charged particles and their attached particles. The collection plates should be cleaned regularly and not be allowed to accumulate large amounts of particulate matter for best operation. Care should be taken if selecting an electrostatic precipitating filter as some varieties generate ozone as their charged particle, which can be irritating to some respiratory patients.

The current U.S. asthma guidelines do not report enough evidence to recommend indoor air cleaning devices across the board. This is based upon the data that suggested that air filtration may reduce some, but not all, airborne allergens and that the true impact on asthma control has not been proven. Specifically, the data has shown that air cleaning devices were useful for removing particles such as airborne dog and cat dander, mold spores, and particulate tobacco smoke. They are not as effective against dust mite and cockroach particles that do not remain airborne for long periods of time. The guidelines also do not make a recommendation on the practice of cleaning air ducts for heating/ventilation/air conditioning systems. They found that there is limited evidence to make a decision one way or another. The EPA agrees that there is currently insufficient information to link air duct cleaning with health benefits. Their indoor air quality Web site provides additional resources on the topic.

Indoor Fungi (Molds)/Sick Building Syndrome

Data has suggested that there is a link between indoor fungi and allergic respiratory disease.[49] The term *sick building syndrome* has been applied to a variety of illnesses attributed to internal environments.[50] Often wet environments and mold growth are attributed to the problems. Each situation is different, and effective management requires a detailed history and diagnosis as well as removal of the mold or irritant. Measures to control dampness or fungal growth in the home environment may be beneficial.[51] The U.S. Environmental Protection Agency (EPA) operates a Web site on indoor air quality that provides resources and more information on sick building syndromes as well as mold, fungi, and other building-related air quality resources.

Radon

Radon is a cancer-causing natural radioactive noble gas that can be found in soil, water, and outdoor and indoor air. It has been estimated that more than 50% of the annual effective dose of natural radioactivity can be attributed to radon exposure. In the United States, radon is the second leading cause of lung cancer (after tobacco smoke) and is believed to claim some 20,000 lives annually.[52] An association between between radon and asthma exacerbations has not been documented.

Useful Web Sites

U.S. Environmental Protection Agency Indoor Air Quality Resources
http://www.epa.gov/iaq/index.html

Should You Have the Air Ducts in Your Home Cleaned?
http://www.epa.gov/iaq/pubs/airduct.html

AIRNOW: Local Air Quality Reports
http://www.airnow.gov/index.cfm?action=airnow.local

Animal/Pet Allergens

Animals release proteins into their surroundings through secretions such as saliva and dander.[53] *Dander* can be defined as organic material or proteins shed from the body of an animal. It has also been called pet pollen. For many allergy sufferers the dander itself may not be irritating, however, it provides an ample food supply for dust mites who are irritating to many asthmatics. Allergens have also been identified in the urine of wild or pet rodents. Ultimately all animals, including humans, provide enough organic dust mite food and bacterial growth opportunities in the home.[54] The current guidelines say that for asthmatics sensitive to animal allergens the treatment of choice is removal of the animal from the home or work environment.[55,56] This is not always practical, as people do love their pets. Asthmatic children will also have friends who have pets and will likely have the opportunity to participate in field trips to the zoo at some time in their school career. It is important that the child and school authorities are made aware of asthmatic risk and are instructed on appropriate responses, should the child begin to develop difficulty. If pets are to remain in the home, they should be kept out of the individual's bedroom and the bedroom door should be kept closed to prevent the pet from entering the area. Upholstered furniture, draperies, and carpets should be removed when possible. If kept in the home, pets should be discouraged from sleeping or lying on the furniture. In addition, regular vacuuming and cleaning of upholstery, draperies, and furniture can also help reduce animal dander buildup and subsequent exposure. It has also been recommended that the pet be washed weekly to minimize potential dander problems. This has not been proven in clinical trials, however.[57] HEPA cleaners have been shown to help reduce airborne *Canis familiaris* allergen 1 (Can f 1) in homes with dogs and decrease the allergen levels in the home.[58] Mice and rodents can also be significant contributors to the dander levels in a home. Pest control that incorporates traps, low-toxicity pesticides, and regular vacuuming and cleaning has been shown to be effective.[1]

Tips for Living with Pets If You Are Asthmatic

- Keep the pet out of the asthmatic's bedroom.
- Keep the bedroom door closed.
- Remove upholstered furniture and carpets from the home, or isolate the pet from these items if possible.
- Wash pillows, plush toys, and linens that the animal comes into contact with regularly (weekly).
- Bathe and brush the pet regularly. (This activity should be done outdoors or away from the asthmatic.)
- Regularly vacuum carpets that the pet has come into contact with (preferably with a HEPA vacuum system).

House Dust Mites

Controlling dust mite allergens is an ongoing battle. Dust mites are unavoidable. Minimizing their impact, however, is manageable. Pillows and mattresses can be encased in plastic allergen covers. Bed linens should be washed weekly in hot water. Using a temperature of >130°F will kill the house dust mites and the washing will reduce their allergens. Pillows can also be washed on a regular basis. Detergents and bleach can also play a significant role in reducing the dust mite allergen in the washing process. Data has shown that cleaning with bleach reduces surface bacteria, airborne fungal spores, and dust antigen levels and improves the quality of life of asthmatics.[59,60] Stuffed animals, toys, and pillows should also be washed weekly to reduce dust mite populations. Prolonged exposure to dry heat or freezing has also been shown to kill mites but does not remove allergens. Dust mites also like a warm wet atmosphere, so decreasing humidity in the home has been suggested as a means to decrease dust mites. Care must be taken, however, to insure that the collection chamber of the dehumidifier is changed frequently and does not become a reservoir for bacterial growth. Sprays and chemical agents are available for killing mites, but their effectiveness is variable and they have not been recommended for routine use.[61] Regular vacuuming is recommended for general cleanliness, but does not remove live dust mites and is not recommended for control of mite allergens.

Cockroach Allergen

Data has shown that cockroach allergen removal and avoidance has a positive impact on asthma outcomes.[62] Food and garbage should not be left out in the home. Poisons, such as cockroach baits and sprays, are effective in managing cockroach infestations, but can be irritating to asthmatics.

Pollen

Pollen season is irritating to many asthmatics. Close monitoring of an individual's asthma care plan during pollen season should be done and adjustments made to their medications as necessary to maintain control. Pollen counts in most parts of the United States peak during the late morning and afternoon. Asthmatics can limit their exposure to these pollens by staying indoors in an air-conditioned environment and keeping the windows closed.[63]

Air Pollution and Traffic Exhaust

Studies have shown that increased particulate matter from traffic exhaust has a negative effect on asthmatics. It is believed that airway oxidative stress increases and small airway function decreases in asthmatics when exposed to air pollution.[64] Many local television stations now provide reports of particulate matter and air quality with the weather reports. The Internet can also provide detailed local reports of air quality. The AirNow Web site, operated as a joint site by several U.S. government agencies, provides state and local level reports with the current air quality index. This index calculates five major air pollutants regulated by the Clean Air Act. These are: ground-level ozone, particle pollution (also known as particulate matter), carbon monoxide, sulfur dioxide, and nitrogen dioxide. The EPA has established national air quality standards for each of these measures and reports the air quality index in comparison to these standards. Asthmatics can limit their exposure by staying indoors in an air-conditioned environment and keeping the windows closed.

Tobacco Smoke

Individuals with asthma, particularly children, should avoid tobacco smoke. Tobacco smoke can precipitate an exacerbation of asthma. Interestingly, the data shows that the effects may vary by age.[65] The effects of second-hand smoke have been shown to be worse on a child's asthma when the mother smokes than when others smoke around them.[66] In addition, studies have shown that maternal smoking increases the risk for the development of asthma in infancy and childhood.[67] Asthmatics and their families should be educated on the avoidance of tobacco smoke and smoke-filled environments.

Aerosolized/Airborne Irritants

Exposure to chemicals such as formaldehyde and volatile organic compounds (VOCs) has been shown to irritate asthmatics' airways and precipitate exacerbations. VOC gases are emitted from a variety of substances such as household products. These include: paints, paint strippers, and other solvents; wood preservatives; aerosol sprays; cleansers and disinfectants; moth repellents;

and air fresheners. The chemicals released into the air by new linoleum flooring, carpeting, wall coverings, furniture, and recent painting have been associated with an increased risk of wheezing in asthmatics.[68] Odors associated with cleaning material, such as bleach and ammonia, may also be irritating to asthmatics as can perfumes, hairsprays, and wood smoke. Individuals with asthma and their families should be counseled on the avoidance of the odors. Unvented gas appliances such as heaters and stoves have been identified as sources of increased levels of NO_2, which increases the risk of wheezing and asthma exacerbations and should be avoided.[69] Exhaust fumes from cars and air pollution, particularly if it is particulate matter of ≤10 micrometers (PM10) in size, have been associated with wheezing and should be avoided.[70,71]

The Hygiene Hypothesis

The hygiene hypothesis has been suggested as an explanation for the rising rates of asthma prevalence. The hypothesis is that our modern emphasis on cleanliness in the western world coupled with the use of vaccinations and antibiotics does not allow the immune system, particularly in children, to fully develop. An immune system that is not stimulated to produce Th1 cells when exposed to microbes will instead create allergy-producing Th2 cells making the individual more likely to develop asthma. The research to date is inconclusive. The hygiene hypothesis is probably not the only explanation for the increased incidence of asthma, but it may be a contributing factor.[72]

What Do All These Types of Asthma Have in Common?

The evidence does show that while the symptoms (i.e., wheezing, shortness of breath, coughing) may vary from individual to individual, airway inflammation is a consistent factor in most cases of true asthma.[73] Fortunately the symptoms of asthma can be controlled and the occurrence of exacerbations decreased and ideally eliminated, if we understand the underlying physiology of the disease.

References

1. Fishman A, et al. *The Biology of Asthma in Fishman's Pulmonary Diseases and Disorders.* Vol. 1. 4th ed. New York: McGraw-Hill Professional; 2008.
2. National Heart, Lung, and Blood Institute. *National Asthma Education and Prevention Program Expert Panel Report 3: Guidelines for the Diagnosis and Management of Asthma Full Report 2007.* http://www.nhlbi.nih.gov/guidelines/asthma/asthsumm.pdf. Accessed April 2, 2009.

3. Lanier BQ, Nayak A. Prevalence and impact of nighttime symptoms in adults and children with asthma: a survey. *Postgrad Med.* 2008;120(4):58–66.
4. Diette GB, Markson L, Skinner EA, Nguyen TT, Algatt-Bergstrom P, Wu AW. Nocturnal asthma in children affects school attendance, school performance, and parents' work attendance. *Arch Pediatr Adolesc Med.* 2000;154(9):923–8.
5. American Academy of Allergy, Asthma, and Immunology. Patients and Consumers: What Is Asthma?: How Can You Tell If Your Child May Have It? March 2000. http://www.aaaai.org/patients/allergic_conditions/pediatric_asthma/what_is_asthma.stm. Accessed on April 24, 2009.
6. American Lung Association. Childhood Asthma Overview. http://www.lungusa.org/site/pp.asp?c=dvLUK9O0E&b=22782#11. Accessed April 24, 2009.
7. Piippo-Savolainen E, Remes S, Kannisto S, Korhonen K, Korppi M. Early predictors for adult asthma and lung function abnormalities in infants hospitalized for bronchiolitis: a prospective 18- to 20-year follow-up. *Allergy Asthma Proc.* 2006;27(4):341–9.
8. Sears MR, Greene JM, Willan AR, Wiecek EM, Taylor DR, Flannery EM, Cowan JO, Herbison GP, Silva PA, Poulton R. A longitudinal, population-based, cohort study of childhood asthma followed to adulthood. *N Engl J Med.* 2003; 349(15):1414–22.
9. Stern DA, Morgan WJ, Halonen M, Wright AL, Martinez FD. Wheezing and bronchial hyperresponsiveness in early childhood as predictors of newly diagnosed asthma in early adulthood: a longitudinal birth-cohort study. *Lancet.* 2008;372(9643):1058–64.
10. Piippo-Savolainen E, Korppi M. Long-term outcomes of early childhood wheezing. *Curr Opin Allergy Clin Immunol.* 2009;9(3):190–6.
11. Piippo-Savolainen E, Korppi M. Wheezy babies—wheezy adults? Review on long-term outcome until adulthood after early childhood wheezing. *Acta Paediatr.* 2008;97(1):5–11.
12. Tarlo S, Balmes J, Balkissoon E, et al. Diagnosis and management of work-related asthma. American College of Chest Physicians Consensus Statement. *Chest.* 2008;134(3):1S–41S.
13. Chan-Yeung M, Malo J-L. Etiologic agents in occupational asthma. *Eur Respir J.* 1994;7:346–371.
14. Dykewicz MS. Occupational asthma: current concepts in pathogenesis, diagnosis, and management. *J Allergy Clin Immunol.* 2009;123(3):519–28; quiz; 529–30.
15. Brooks SM, Weiss MA, Bernstein IL. Reactive airways dysfunction syndrome (RADS). Persistent asthma syndrome after high level irritant exposure. *Chest.* 1985;88:376–384.
16. Alberts WM, do Pico GA. Reactive airways dysfunction syndrome. *Chest.* 1996;109:1618–1626.
17. Mapp CE, Miotto D, Boschetto P. Occupational asthma. *Med Lav.* 2006; 97(2):404–9.
18. American Lung Association. Occupational asthma. http://www.lungusa.org/site/pp.asp?c=dvLUK9O0E&b=22597. Accessed April 24, 2009.
19. Diette GB, Markson L, Skinner EA, et al. Nocturnal asthma in children affects school attendance, school performance, and parents' work attendance. *Arch Pediatr Adolesc Med.* 2000;154:923–928.

20. Avidan B, Sonnenberg A, Schnell TG, Sontag SJ. Temporal associations between coughing or wheezing and acid reflux in asthmatics. *Gut*. 2001;49(6):767–72.
21. Littner MR, Leung FW, Ballard ED, et al. Effects of 24 weeks of lansoprazole therapy on asthma symptoms, exacerbations, quality of life, and pulmonary function in adult asthmatic patients with acid reflux symptoms. *Chest*. 2005;128(3):1128–35.
22. Alkhalil M, Schulman E, Getsy J. Obstructive sleep apnea syndrome and asthma: what are the links? *J Clin Sleep Med*. 2009;5(1):71–8.
23. Alkhalil M, Schulman ES, Getsy J. Obstructive sleep apnea syndrome and asthma: the role of continuous positive airway pressure treatment. *Ann Allergy Asthma Immunol*. 2008;101(4):350–7.
24. Ciftci TU, Ciftci B, Guven SF, Kokturk O, Turktas H. Effect of nasal continuous positive airway pressure in uncontrolled nocturnal asthmatic patients with obstructive sleep apnea syndrome. *Respir Med*. 2005;99(5):529–34. Epub: November 23, 2004.
25. Rundell KW, Jenkinson DM. Exercise-induced bronchospasm in the elite athlete. *Sports Med*. 2002;32:583–600.
26. Parsons JP, Mastronarde JG. Exercise-induced bronchoconstriction in athletes. *Chest*. 2005;128(6):3966–74.
27. Hurwitz KM, Argyros GJ, Roach JM, et al. Interpretation of eucapnic voluntary hyperventilation in the diagnosis of asthma. *Chest*. 1995;108:1240–1245.
28. Schatz M, Harden K, Forsythe A, Chilingar L, Hoffman C, Sperling W, et al. The course of asthma during pregnancy, post partum, and with successive pregnancies: a prospective analysis. *J Allergy Clin Immunol*. 1988;81(3):509–17.
29. Schatz M. Interrelationships between asthma and pregnancy: a literature review. *J Allergy Clin Immunol*. 1999;103(2;2):S330–6.
30. Demissie K, Breckenridge MB, Rhoads GG. Infant and maternal outcomes in the pregnancies of asthmatic women. *Am J Respir Crit Care Med*. 1998;158(4):1091–5.
31. Chien S, Mintz S. Pregnancy and menses. In: Weiss EB, Stein M, eds. *Bronchial Asthma Mechanisms and Therapeutics*. Boston: Little Brown; 1993.
32. Ito K, Chung KF, Adcock IM. Update on glucocorticoid action and resistance. *J Allergy Clin Immunol*. 2006;117(3):522–43.
33. Wenzel SE. Asthma: defining of the persistent adult phenotypes. *Lancet*. 2006;368(9537):804–13.
34. Ito K, Chung KF, Adcock IM. Update on glucocorticoid action and resistance. *J Allergy Clin Immunol*. 2006;117(3):522–43.
35. Barnes PJ, Adcock IM, Ito K. Histone acetylation and deacetylation: importance in inflammatory lung diseases. *Eur Respir J*. 2005;25:552–563.
36. Szczeklik A, Stevenson DD. Aspirin-induced asthma: advances in pathogenesis, diagnosis, and management. *J Allergy Clin Immunol*. 2003;111(5):913–21.
37. Spector SL, Wangaard CH, Farr RS. Aspirin and concomitant idiosyncrasies in adult asthmatic patients. *J Allergy Clin Immunol*. 1979;64(6;1):500–6.
38. Stevenson DD. Aspirin sensitivity and desensitization for asthma and sinusitis. *Curr Allergy Asthma Rep*. 2009;9(2):155–63.
39. Szczeklik A, Sanak M. Genetic mechanisms in aspirin-induced asthma. *Am J Respir Crit Care Med*. 2000;161(2;2):S142–6.

40. Dahlen SE, Malmstrom K, Nizankowska E, Dahlen B, Kuna P, Kowalski M, et al. Improvement of aspirin-intolerant asthma by montelukast, a leukotriene antagonist: a randomized, double-blind, placebo-controlled trial. *Am J Respir Crit Care Med.* 2002;165(1):9–14.
41. Nizankowska E, Bestynska-Krypel A, Cmiel A, Szczeklik A. Oral and bronchial provocation tests with aspirin for diagnosis of aspirin-induced asthma. *Eur Respir J.* 2000;15(5):863–9.
42. Simon RA. Adverse respiratory reactions to aspirin and nonsteroidal anti-inflammatory drugs. *Curr Allergy Asthma Rep.* 2004;4(1):17–24.
43. Stevenson DD. Aspirin desensitization in patients with AERD. *Clin Rev Allergy Immunol.* 2003;24(2):159–68.
44. Jain S, Bandi V, Officer T, Wolley M, Guntupalli KK. Role of vocal cord function and dysfunction in patients presenting with symptoms of acute asthma exacerbation. *J Asthma.* 2006;43(3):207–212.
45. King CS, Moores LK. Clinical asthma syndromes and important asthma mimics. *Respir Care.* 2008;53(5):568–80; discussion:580–2.
46. Ibrahim WH, Gheriani HA, Almohamed AA, Raza T. Paradoxical vocal cord motion disorder: past, present and future. *Postgrad Med J.* 2007;83(977):164–72.
47. Boyce JA, Broide D, Matsumoto K, Bochner BS. Advances in mechanisms of asthma, allergy, and immunology in 2008. *J Allergy Clin Immunol.* 2009;123(3):569–74.
48. Mason RJ, Broaddus VC, Murray JF, et al. *Murray and Nadel's Textbook of Respiratory Medicine.* Vol. 1. 4th ed. Philadelphia: W.B. Saunders; 2005.
49. Bjornsson E, Norback D, Janson C, Widstrom J, Palmgren U, Strom G, Boman G. Asthmatic symptoms and indoor levels of micro-organisms and house dust mites. *Clin Exp Allergy.* 1995;25(5):423–31.
50. Jaakkola MS, Jaakkola JJ. Office work exposures and adult-onset asthma. *J Environ Health Perspect.* 2007;115(7):1007–11.
51. Hope AP, Simon RA. Excess dampness and mold growth in homes: an evidence-based review of the aeroirritant effect and its potential causes. *Allergy Asthma Proc.* 2007;28(3):262–70.
52. Al-Zoughool M, Krewski D. Health effects of radon: a review of the literature. *Int J Radiat Biol.* 2009;85(1):57–69.
53. Erwin EA, Woodfolk JA, Custis N, Platts-Mills TA. Animal danders. *Immunol Allergy Clin North Am.* 2003;23(3):469–81.
54. Erwin EA, Woodfolk JA, Custis N, Platts-Mills TA. Animal danders. *Immunol Allergy Clin North Am.* 2003;23(3):469–81.
55. National Heart, Lung, and Blood Institute. National Asthma Education and Prevention Program Expert Panel Report 3: Guidelines for the Diagnosis and Management of Asthma Full Report 2007. http://www.nhlbi.nih.gov/guidelines/asthma/asthsumm.pdf. Accessed April 2, 2009.
56. The Global Initiative for Asthma (GINA). 2009 update of the GINA Report, Global Strategy for Asthma Management and Prevention. http://www.ginasthma.com. Accessed April 1, 2010.
57. Avner DB, Perzanowski MS, Platts-Mills TA, Woodfolk JA. Evaluation of different techniques for washing cats: quantitation of allergen removed from the cat and the effect on airborne Fel d 1. *J Allergy Clin Immunol.* 1997;100(3):307–12.

58. Green R, Simpson A, Custovic A, Faragher B, Chapman M, Woodcock A. The effect of air filtration on airborne dog allergen. *Allergy*. 1999;54(5):484–8.
59. Barnes CS, Kennedy K, Gard L, et al. The impact of home cleaning on quality of life for homes with asthmatic children. *Allergy Asthma Proc*. 2008;29(2):197–204.
60. Arlian LG, Vyszenski-Moher DL, Morgan MS. Mite and mite allergen removal during machine washing of laundry. *J Allergy Clin Immunol*. 2003;111(6):1269–73.
61. Klucka CV, Ownby DR, Green J, Zoratti E. Cat shedding of Fel d I is not reduced by washings, Allerpet-C spray, or acepromazine. *J Allergy Clin Immunol*. 1995; 95(6):1164–71.
62. Morgan WJ, Crain EF, Gruchalla RS, O'Connor GT, Kattan M, Evans R III, Stout J, Malindzak G, Smartt E, Plaut M, et al. Inner-City Asthma Study Group. Results of a home-based environmental intervention among urban children with asthma. *N Engl J Med*. 2004;351(11):1068–80.
63. Lierl MB, Hornung RW. Relationship of outdoor air quality to pediatric asthma exacerbations. *Ann Allergy Asthma Immunol*. 2003;90(1):28–33.
64. Liu L, Poon R, Chen L, et al. Acute effects of air pollution on pulmonary function, airway inflammation, and oxidative stress in asthmatic children. *Environ Health Perspect*. 2009;117(4):668–74.
65. Mannino DM, Moorman JE, Kingsley B, Rose D, Repace J. Health effects related to environmental tobacco smoke exposure in children in the United States: data from the Third National Health and Nutrition Examination Survey. *Arch Pediatr Adolesc Med*. 2001;155(1):36–41.
66. Agabiti N, Mallone S, Forastiere F, Corbo GM, Ferro S, Renzoni E, Sestini P, Rusconi F, Ciccone G, Viegi G, et al. The impact of parental smoking on asthma and wheezing. SIDRIA Collaborative Group. Studi Italiani sui Disturbi Respiratori nell'Infanzia e l'Ambiente. *Epidemiol*. 1999;10(6):692–8.
67. Martinez FD, Wright AL, Taussig LM, Holberg CJ, Halonen M, Morgan WJ. Asthma and wheezing in the first six years of life. The Group Health Medical Associates. *N Engl J Med*. 1995;332(3):133–8.
68. Jaakkola JJ, Parise H, Kislitsin V, Lebedeva NI, Spengler JD. Asthma, wheezing, and allergies in Russian schoolchildren in relation to new surface materials in the home. *Am J Public Health*. 2004;94(4):560–2.
69. Garrett MH, Hooper MA, Hooper BM, Abramson MJ. Respiratory symptoms in children and indoor exposure to nitrogen dioxide and gas stoves. *Am J Respir Crit Care Med*. 1998;158(3):891–5.
70. Atkinson RW, Anderson HR, Sunyer J, Ayres J, Baccini M, Vonk JM, Boumghar A, Forastiere F, Forsberg B, Touloumi G, et al. Acute effects of particulate air pollution on respiratory admissions: results from APHEA 2 project. Air Pollution and Health: a European Approach. *Am J Respir Crit Care Med*. 2001;164(10;1):1860–6.
71. Gent JF, Triche EW, Holford TR, Belanger K, Bracken MB, Beckett WS, Leaderer BP. Association of low-level ozone and fine particles with respiratory symptoms in children with asthma. *JAMA*. 2003;290(14):1859–67.
72. Ramsey CD, Celedón JC. The hygiene hypothesis and asthma. *Curr Opin Pulm Med*. 2005;11(1):14–20.
73. The Global Initiative for Asthma (GINA). 2009 Update of the GINA Report, Global Strategy for Asthma Management and Prevention. http://www.ginasthma.com. Accessed April 1, 2010.

3

The Pathophysiology of Asthma

LEARNING OBJECTIVES

- Review the components of airflow limitation
- Discuss the inflammatory cascade in asthma
- Identify the pathways to asthma control

KEY WORDS

bronchoconstriction
airway edema
airway hyperresponsiveness
airway inflammation
eosinophils
chemokines
cysteinyl leukotrienes
lymphocytes
$CD4^+$ T cells
interleukins
tumor necrosis factor (TNF)
granulocyte macrophage-colony stimulating factor (GM-CSF)
immunoglobulin (Ig)
interferon (IFN)

The Pathophysiology of Asthma

The pathophysiological features of asthma are airflow limitation and airway inflammation.[1] Understanding these mechanisms within the airway provides a roadmap to developing successful treatment plans and gaining/maintaining asthma control.

Airflow Limitation/Airway Narrowing

The exact etiology of airflow limitation in asthma is still unknown, though several factors have been linked to the occurrence. A common component is bronchial smooth muscle contraction (bronchoconstriction), which is defined as the rapid contraction or narrowing of the airway in response to bronchoconstrictor mediators and neurotransmitters.[2] It is this airway narrowing that leads to airflow limitation and produces the "wheeze" so often associated with asthma. Bronchoconstriction is largely reversed by bronchodilators. Airway edema or fluid in the airway is caused by microvascular leakage in response to inflammatory mediators. This may be reversible by anti-inflammatory medications. *Mucus hypersecretion* is the term applied to the increased mucus secretion and inflammatory exudates that occur in asthma. Data has shown that an increased number of goblet cells in the airway epithelium and increased size of submucosal glands occur in asthma. Mucous plugging is said to occur when a portion of the airway becomes clogged and air is not able to move in and out of the airways below. Airway remodeling refers to structural changes of the airway that occur over time. We do know that even before the onset of symptoms, many asthma patients have some degree of airway remodeling. Subepithelial fibrosis occurs as a result of collagen fibers and proteoglycans forming under the basement membrane. These substances can also deposit in other layers for the airway wall causing fibrosis in those areas. The airway's smooth muscle increases in size due to two primary mechanisms: hypertrophy (increased size of individual cells) and hyperplasia (increased cell division).[2] This results in an increased thickness of the airway wall.[3] It is believed that inflammatory mediators play a role in these changes. We also know that there is an increased proliferation of blood vessels in airway walls that may contribute to increased airway wall thickness as well. Data has shown that these changes are associated with the severity of the patient's asthma and is not fully reversible by current therapy.[4]

Components of Airflow Limitation/Airway Narrowing

- Bronchial smooth muscle contraction (bronchoconstriction)
- Airway edema
- Mucus hypersecretion
- Airway remodeling (hypertrophy and hyperplasia)

Adapted from: The Global Initiative for Asthma (GINA). 2009 Update of the GINA Report, Global Strategy for Asthma Management and Prevention. http://www.ginasthma.com. Accessed April 12, 2010.

Airway Hyperresponsiveness

Airway hyperresponsiveness is the term used to describe the tendency of the airways to narrow in response to exposure to a variety of stimuli. As we will see in the chapter on diagnosis, airway hyperresponsiveness is quantified by the degree of contractile responses to a methacholine challenge test, which helps determine the clinical severity of the individual's asthma.

Bronchoconstriction or Airway Hyperresponsiveness: What Is the Difference?

- *Bronchoconstriction* is the actual mechanical contraction of the airway.
- *Airway hyperresponsiveness* is the likelihood or chance that it is going to contract and to what degree.

Airway Inflammation

Data has shown that airway inflammation occurs in asthma even when airway limitation symptoms are not present.[5] It also occurs regardless of the type of asthma (allergic vs. nonallergic). Though usually called airway inflammation, it occurs throughout the respiratory system. However, it seems to have the most impact on the medium-sized bronchi. The inflammation associated with asthma follows the same pattern as inflammation occurring in an allergic response. The following subsections detail the major components of airway inflammation.

Immunoglobulin

Immunoglobulin (Ig) is a small protein molecule created by the immune system to "fit" onto the surface of the antigen or irritant. By attaching themselves to the surface of the antigen they serve as flags to call the rest of the immune system cells to come and help fight the invader. There are a complex series of events that lead up to the production of Ig. When an antigen enters the body, a specific type of white blood cell known as a T lymphocyte, or T cell, arrives at the antigen site and determines what is needed to fight the invader. The T cell uses "helper" cells, also known as TH cells, to direct the release of cytokines that stimulate the B lymphocytes. The B lymphocytes are the cells that actually produce the Ig antibodies that bind to the antigen. The term *B-cell proliferation* is used once an Ig has bound with an antigen and triggered the B lymphocyte to reproduce and make more Ig.[6] TH cells are believed to always express the surface protein CD4, therefore they are also known as $CD4^+$ T cells.

There are several classes of antibodies elicited by an allergic trigger also known as immunoglobulins (Ig). Among these are: IgM, IgG, IgA, IgD, and IgE. When specifically discussing an allergy, including allergic asthma, IgE is the immunoglobulin involved. When the body responds to an antigen by specifically producing IgE, the antigen is called an allergen and the individual is said to have had atopy or allergies. In these individuals, IgE has been found circulating in the blood along with inflammatory cells called basophils and bound to the surface of inflammatory cells throughout the body known as mast cells.[6]

Mast Cells and Basophils

Basophils are found in the bloodstream. Mast cells are found in many tissues of the body, particularly the airway tissue. Both of these inflammatory cells have over 100,000 receptor sites each for IgE. When an individual is exposed to an allergen and produces IgE that binds to these receptor sites, these mast cells and basophils are said to be *primed*. The next time the individual is exposed to that allergen the mast cells and basophils will release chemical mediators that cause the allergic response. Clinicians should note that once sensitized, mast cells and basophils can remain primed for months or even years.[6]

Chemical Mediators

The best known chemical mediator released by the mast cells is histamine. Histamine attaches to the histamine receptors (H1) that can be found in most cells of the body and stimulate allergic symptoms such as swelling, sneezing, and itching. Another family of chemical mediators is the *cysteinyl leukotrienes*. These substances are usually released between 5 and 30 minutes after activation of the mast cells or basophils. While they have the same basic effect as histamine, they are usually more potent. Specifically, Leukotriene D4 is 10 times more potent than histamine.[6] The cysteinyl leukotrienes are the only mediators whose inhibition has been associated with improvements in asthma symptoms and pulmonary function values.[7] Another family of mediators, known as *chemokines*, are expressed in airway epithelial cells and are responsible for the recruitment of inflammatory cells into the airways. Eotaxin is a chemokine that is relatively selective for eosinophil recruitment. Thymus and activation-regulated chemokines (TARC) and macrophage-derived chemokines (MDC) have been shown to recruit Th2 cells.[8]

Cytokines are signaling proteins that provide cellular communication during the inflammatory response in asthma. Measuring their levels can help determine the severity of the inflammatory response. They can be divided into four categories: lymphokines are cytokines that are produced by T lymphocytes; proinflammatory cytokines amplify and carry on the inflammatory response; anti-inflammatory cytokines inhibit inflammation; and chemokines were discussed in the preceding paragraph. Regulation of cytokines in airway cells is one of the major targets of corticosteroid therapy and T-cell immunosuppressants in asthma. See Table 3.1 for some common cytokines that occur in asthma.

Nitric oxide (NO) is a potent vasodilator that is produced in airway epithelial cells. NO plays a role in the regulation of vascular tone, response to vascular injury, and hemostasis. It is a neurotransmitter for the nonadrenergic noncholinergic nerves and also has antimicrobial, immunologic, and proinflammatory activities. Exhaled NO is increased during bronchospasm with coexisting inflammation. Therefore the measurement of exhaled NO is a noninvasive test for the evaluation of inflammation associated with asthma and has been used as a marker for determining the effectiveness of asthma treatment.[9]

TABLE 3.1 Some Common Cytokines That Occur in Asthma and Their Function

Lymphokines	
IL-2	Stimulates growth and differentiation of T cells
IL-4	Proinflammatory yet classified as a lymphokine Crucial for the development of Th2 cells and for IgE synthesis from B cells
IL-5	Triggers eosinophilic inflammation
IL-13	Activates eosinophils, increases IgE production
Proinflammatory Cytokines	
TNF-α	Expressed in asthmatic airways and may be important in amplifying asthmatic inflammation
IL-6	Promotes IgE synthesis
GM-CSF	Stimulates eosinophils and the release of leukotrienes
Anti-Inflammatory Cytokines	
IL-10	A potent anti-inflammatory cytokine that inhibits the synthesis of many inflammatory proteins, including cytokines
IFN-y	Inhibits Th2 cells and reduces atopic inflammation
IL-12	Stimulates the development of Th1 cells, while suppressing the occurrence of Th2 cells

IL = interleukins; TNF = tumor necrosis factor; GM-CSF = granulocyte macrophage-colony stimulating factor; Th = helper T lymphocytes; IgE = immunoglobulin; IFN = interferon

Adapted from: Chung KF, Barnes PJ. Cytokines in asthma. *Thorax.*1999; 54(9):825–57. Doshi U, Salat P, Parikh V. Cytokine modulators in asthma: clinical perspectives. *Indian J Pharmacol.* 2002;34:16–25.

Prostaglandin D2

Prostaglandin D2 is a potent bronchoconstrictor involved in Th2 cell recruitment to the airways. Prostaglandin D2 is derived for the most part from the mast cells.[2]

Airway Inflammation: The Actual Process

Now that we know the players we can address the process. When an allergen or asthma trigger enters the airway the mast and the Th2 cells in the airway are activated. They induce the production of mediators such as histamine, leukotrienes, and cytokines. The mediators go to work alerting the immune system and recruiting help to combat the invader. Inflammation in the form of swelling of the bronchial wall coupled with increases in bronchial secretions occurs in response to these cytokines' activities (see Figure 3.1).

Pathways to Controlling Asthma

If we think of asthma as a two component disease (airflow limitation and airway inflammation), the current strategies for managing asthma becomes much easier. Current management strategies employ a reliever medication for the reversal of acute airflow limitation (bronchoconstriction) and controller medications that prevent airway inflammation from happening. As professionals we understand that this is not as physiologically cut and dried as it seems—there are some overlapping mechanisms between airflow limitation and airway inflammation. But, it is an effective tool not only to assist our understanding when developing a treatment plan, but to help patients understand why both types of medication are important. Or in a nutshell: *asthma is a dual component disease so it requires a dual medication strategy*.

Genetics and Asthma

The mapping of the human genome has led to an explosion in the potential candidate genes for asthma and atopy. Complicating the matter is that we now classify asthma as a disease of both airway hyperresponsiveness and inflammation making both of these pathways candidates for a genetic origin of asthma.[10] Specifically, genes found on the cytokine gene cluster of chromosome 5 (for example, the genes relating to interleukin-3, -4, -5, -9, and -13), chromosome 11 (the beta chain of the high-affinity IgE receptor), chromosome 16 (the IL-4 receptor), and chromosome 12 (stem cell factor, interferon-gamma, insulin growth factor, and Stat 6 [IL-4 Stat]) have all been implicated in asthma.[11] It is likely no one single asthma gene will be

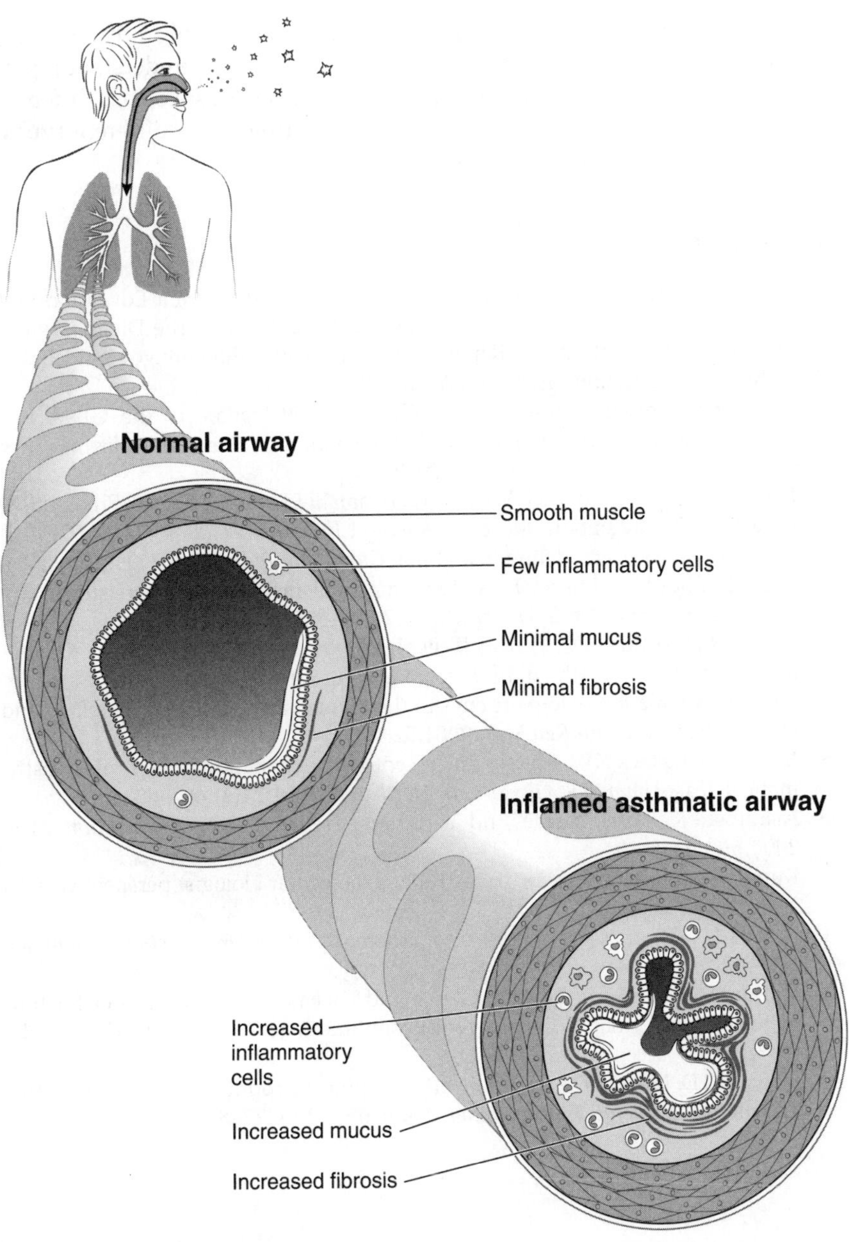

FIGURE 3.1 Pathways to controlling asthma.

identified. It is hoped that by focusing on the identified chromosomes further genes will be identified that will lead to an improved understanding of pathogenic factors and treatment options. It is also possible that different gene combinations may be identified as contributing to the different types, severities, and/or triggers of asthma.[12,13]

References

1. National Heart, Lung, and Blood Institute. National Asthma Education and Prevention Program Expert Panel Report 3: Guidelines for the Diagnosis and Management of Asthma Full Report 2007. http://www.nhlbi.nih.gov/guidelines/asthma/asthsumm.pdf. Accessed April 2, 2009.
2. The Global Initiative for Asthma (GINA). 2009 Update of the GINA Report, Global Strategy for Asthma Management and Prevention. http://www.ginasthma.com. Accessed April 1, 2010.
3. Hirst SJ, Martin JG, Bonacci JV, Chan V, Fixman ED, Hamid QA, et al. Proliferative aspects of airway smooth muscle. *J Allergy Clin Immunol.* 2004;114(2):S2–17.
4. James A. Airway remodeling in asthma. *Curr Opin Pulm Med.* 2005;11(1):1–6.
5. Cohn L, Elias JA, Chupp GL. Asthma: mechanisms of disease persistence and progression. *Annu Rev Immunol.* 2004;22:789–815.
6. Mason RJ, Broaddus VC, Murray JF, et al. *Murray and Nadel's Textbook of Respiratory Medicine.* Vol 1. 4th ed. Philadelphia: W.B. Saunders; 2005.
7. Leff AR. Regulation of leukotrienes in the management of asthma: biology and clinical therapy. *Annu Rev Med.* 2001;52:1–14.
8. Miller AL, Lukacs NW. Chemokine receptors: understanding their role in asthmatic disease. *Immunol Allergy Clin North Am.* 2004;24(4):667–83.
9. Ashutosh K. Nitric oxide and asthma: a review. *Curr Opin Pulm Med.* 2000;6(1):21–5.
10. Kumar A, Ghosh B, Genetics of asthma: a molecular biologist perspective. *Clin Mol Allergy.* 2009;7:7.
11. Borish L. Genetics of allergy and asthma. *Ann Allergy Asthma Immunol.* 1999;82(5):413–24;
12. National Institutes of Health. Genes and Disease; National Center for Biotechnology Information. http://www.ncbi.nlm.nih.gov/books/bv.fcgi?rid=gnd&ref=sidebar. Accessed July 17, 2009.
13. Howard TD, Meyers DA, Bleecker ER. Mapping susceptibility genes for asthma and allergy. *J Allergy Clin Immunol.* 2000;105(2;2):S477–81.

4 Diagnosing Asthma

LEARNING OBJECTIVES

- Review the methods to assess airflow limitation and diagnose asthma
- Discuss the interaction between lung volume and patients' symptoms
- Identify the criteria for referral to an asthma specialist

KEY WORDS

spirometry
forced expiratory volume in 1 second (FEV_1)
forced vital capacity (FVC)
peak expiratory flow (PEF)
airway responsiveness
methacholine challenge
dyspnea
hyperextension
differential diagnosis

Diagnosing Asthma

The intermittent nature and wide variation in asthma symptoms make diagnosing the condition a challenge. Yet, proper diagnosis is essential to assuring appropriate treatment and management of asthma. Individuals presenting with breathlessness, wheezing, cough, and chest tightness should be considered as potential asthmatics; however, this symptomatology is not exclusive to asthma. A variety of conditions can mimic asthma and should be ruled out. Some alternative causes of recurrent wheezing that must be considered and excluded are described in Table 4.1.

TABLE 4.1 Some Causes of Recurrent Wheezing

Chronic rhinosinusitis
Chronic obstructive pulmonary disease
Bronchiectasis
Gastroesophageal reflux
Recurrent viral lower respiratory tract infections
Cystic fibrosis
Bronchopulmonary dysplasia
Tuberculosis
Congenital malformation causing narrowing of the intrathoracic airways
Foreign body aspiration
Primary ciliary dyskinesia syndrome
Immune deficiency
Congenital heart disease
Prematurity in neonates
Neonatal onset of symptoms associated with failure to thrive
Hyperventilation syndrome and panic attacks

Adapted from: The Global Initiative for Asthma (GINA). 2009 Update of the GINA Report, Global Strategy for Asthma Management and Prevention. http://www.ginasthma.com. Accessed April 1, 2010.[1]

Realistically screening every individual for asthma is neither practical nor is it the best use of resources. A simple questionnaire however can help identify individuals that are at risk and may be having mild asthma symptoms (see Table 4.2). The questionnaire can be included in the initial paperwork that the individual fills out in a physicians' office or upon admission to the hospital. There are a variety of versions of the questionnaire, including one available from the American Lung Association and also in the current asthma guidelines. The most common name for this type of screening is the Asthma Symptom Score/Scale. Answering yes to any one of the questions is suggestive of a risk for asthma and should be further evaluated.

Additional questions may be added to the asthma score dependent upon your patient population. For example you may wish to add a question related to allergens or irritants if you live in a location that has a particular problem with these. If you are seeing primarily school age children you may wish to add more questions about exercise-related symptoms. If individuals answer yes to any of these questions, they should be further assessed for asthma (see Table 4.3).

TABLE 4.2 Asthma Symptom Score/Scale

In the past 12 months …	*Scoring: Yes = 1, No = 0*
Have you had a sudden severe episode or recurrent episodes of coughing, wheezing (high-pitched whistling sounds when breathing out), chest tightness, or shortness of breath?	
Have you had colds that "go to the chest" or take more than 10 days to get over?	
Have you had coughing, wheezing, or shortness of breath during a particular season or time of the year?	
Have you had coughing, wheezing, or shortness of breath in certain places or when exposed to certain things (e.g., animals, tobacco smoke, perfumes)?	
Have you used any medications that help you breathe better? How often?	
Are your symptoms relieved when the medications are used?	
In the past 4 weeks, have you had coughing, wheezing, or shortness of breath …	
At night that has awakened you?	
Upon awakening?	
After running, moderate exercise, or other physical activity?	
Total Score	

Adapted from: National Heart, Lung, and Blood Institute. National Asthma Education and Prevention Program Expert Panel Report 3: Guidelines for the Diagnosis and Management of Asthma Full Report 2007. http://www.nhlbi.nih.gov/guidelines/asthma/asthsumm.pdf. Accessed April 2, 2009.[2]

TABLE 4.3 How to Establish a Diagnosis of Asthma

1. Take a detailed medical history.
2. Conduct a physical exam focusing on the upper respiratory tract, chest, and skin.
3. Perform spirometry to demonstrate obstruction and assess reversibility.
4. Perform additional testing as necessary to exclude other diagnosis such as chronic obstructive pulmonary disease (COPD), vocal chord dysfunction (VCD), etc.

Adapted from: National Heart, Lung, and Blood Institute. National Asthma Education and Prevention Program Expert Panel Report 3: Guidelines for the Diagnosis and Management of Asthma Full Report 2007. http://www.nhlbi.nih.gov/guidelines/asthma/asthsumm.pdf. Accessed April 2, 2009.[2]

Medical History

A complete medical history is essential to properly diagnosing asthma. It can also be suggestive of the individual's asthma severity and likelihood to experience an exacerbation. Data has shown that exacerbations that require emergency department (ED) visits, hospitalization, or intensive care unit (ICU) stays increase the individual's risk of having another serious episode. This risk is also increased if the event happened in the last year.[3,4] When taking a medical history it is important to identify not only the potential asthma symptoms, but also what may have precipitated them. Ideally you are trying to establish that there is an episodic occurrence of airflow obstruction or airway hyperresponsiveness that it is at least partially reversible, and that you have ruled out all other alternative diagnoses. The easiest way to do this is to identify the symptoms that may or may not be asthma and then look for patterns of the symptoms either in the individuals or in their family history. An example of the information that could be asked in a medical history is provided in Table 4.4.

TABLE 4.4 Suggested Items for a Medical History*

1. Symptoms	• Cough • Wheezing • Shortness of breath • Chest tightness • Sputum production
2. Pattern of symptoms	• Perennial, seasonal, or both • Continual, episodic, or both • Onset, duration, frequency (number of days or nights, per week or month) • Diurnal variations, especially nocturnal and on awakening in early morning
3. Precipitating and/or aggravating factors	• Viral respiratory infections • Environmental allergens, indoor (e.g., mold, house dust mite, cockroach, animal dander, or animal/insect secretory products) and outdoor (e.g., pollen) • Characteristics of home including age, location, cooling and heating system, wood-burning stove, humidifier, carpeting over concrete, presence of molds or mildew, characteristics of rooms where patient spends time (e.g., bedroom and living room with attention to bedding, floor covering, stuffed furniture) • Smoking (patient and others in home or daycare)

TABLE 4.4 Suggested Items for a Medical History *(Cont.)*

	• Exercise • Occupational chemicals or allergens • Environmental change (e.g., moving to new home; going on vacation; alterations in workplace, work processes, or materials used) • Irritants (e.g., tobacco smoke, strong odors, air pollutants, occupational chemicals, dusts and particulates, vapors, gases, and aerosols) • Emotions (e.g., fear, anger, frustration, hard crying, or laughing) • Stress (e.g., fear, anger, frustration) • Drugs (e.g., aspirin and other NSAIDs, beta-blockers including eye drops) • Food, food additives, and preservatives (e.g., sulfites) • Changes in weather, exposure to cold air • Endocrine factors (e.g., menses, pregnancy, thyroid disease) • Comorbid conditions (e.g., sinusitis, rhinitis, GERD)
4. Development of disease and treatment	• Age of onset and diagnosis • History of early-life injury to airways (e.g., bronchopulmonary dysplasia, pneumonia, parental smoking) • Progression of disease (better or worse) • Present management and response, including plans for managing exacerbations • Frequency of using rescue medication • Need for oral corticosteroids and frequency of use
5. Family history	• History of asthma, allergy, sinusitis, rhinitis, eczema, or nasal polyps in close relatives
6. Social history	• Daycare, workplace, and school characteristics that may interfere with adherence • Social factors that interfere with adherence, such as substance abuse • Social support/social networks • Level of education completed • Employment

(continues)

TABLE 4.4 Suggested Items for a Medical History *(Cont.)*

7. History of exacerbations	• Usual prodromal signs and symptoms • Rapidity of onset • Duration • Frequency • Severity (need for urgent care, hospitalization, ICU admission) • Life-threatening exacerbations (e.g., intubation, intensive care unit admission) • Number and severity of exacerbations in the past year • Usual patterns and management (what works?)
8. Impact of asthma on patient and family	• Episodes of unscheduled care (ED, urgent care, hospitalization) • Number of days missed from school/work • Limitation of activity, especially sports and strenuous work • History of nocturnal awakening • Effect on growth, development, behavior, school or work performance, and lifestyle • Impact on family routines, activities, or dynamics • Economic impact
9. Assessment of patient's and family's perceptions of disease	• Patient's, parents', and spouse's or partner's knowledge of asthma and belief in the chronicity of asthma and in the efficacy of treatment • Patient's perception and beliefs regarding use and long-term effects of medications • Ability of patient and parents, spouse, or partner to cope with disease • Level of family support and patient's and parents', spouse's, or partner's capacity to recognize severity of an exacerbation • Economic resources • Sociocultural beliefs

*This list does not represent a standardized assessment or diagnostic instrument. The validity and reliability of this list have not been assessed.

Adapted from National Heart, Lung, and Blood Institute. National Asthma Education and Prevention Program Expert Panel Report 3: Guidelines for the Diagnosis and Management of Asthma Full Report 2007. http://www.nhlbi.nih.gov/guidelines/asthma/asthsumm.pdf. Accessed April 2, 2009.[2]

Physical Exam Focusing on the Upper Respiratory Tract, Chest, and Skin

When conducting a physical exam the usual vital signs (e.g., heart rate, blood pressure, temperature) should be noted; they do not directly relate to asthma, but can give clues to the individual's overall health. Examination of the upper airway should include an assessment of any sinus or allergy symptoms the individual may be experiencing. The presence of increased nasal secretion, mucosal swelling, and/or nasal polyps should be noted and evaluated for allergy-related asthma. Examination of the chest includes assessment of breath sounds. The presence of wheezing, defined as high-pitched whistling sound during exhalation, is suggestive of asthma. Practitioners should note that the wheezing may only be heard with a stethoscope or not at all. The absence of wheezing during the examination does not mean the individual does not have asthma, it just means they are not symptomatic at that time. If other factors suggest that they may have asthma, test further. Respiratory rate and rhythm should also be assessed as should chest wall expansion. Hyperexpansion of the chest, use of the accessory muscles for breathing, or a hunched appearance is suggestive of a respiratory problem. Examination of the skin is also recommended. Specifically, the presence of atopic dermatitis or a rash suggests that there is an allergic component that may be at work.

Chest radiographs (X-rays) and pulse oximetry, in and of themselves, are not diagnostic tests for asthma. They can be useful tools for providing more information to the individual's overall health. If the patient's history and physical examination are suggestive of asthma, the next diagnostic step is pulmonary function studies.

Spirometry Versus Peak Flow Monitoring

Both spirometry and peak flow measurement are useful and necessary for asthma control.

Spirometry is diagnostic and can provide a snapshot of the smaller airway function.

Peak flow measurement is useful for monitoring and measures larger airway function.

Pulmonary Function Studies

Pulmonary function studies measure the volume of air going in and out of the lungs, the speed at which that air moves in and out, and the volume of the air that is moving. An objective pulmonary function study can not only diagnose asthma, but can rule out or identify other respiratory diseases that may be present.

A basic pulmonary function study, also known as spirometry, includes a variety of tests. The forced vital capacity test (FVC) measures the maximal volume of air forcibly exhaled from the point of maximal inhalation and the volume of air exhaled during the first second of this maneuver; this is known as the FEV_1. A slow vital capacity (SVC) is often coupled with an FVC to verify the volume measurements. Ideally, the volume numbers should be the same in both the FVC and the SVC. However, signs of airflow limitation may be present and include reduced FEV_1 and a reduced FEV_1/FVC ratio. The FVC may be decreased as a result of air trapping. Overall, lung volume measurements may show an increase in the residual volume, the functional residual capacity, or both

Pre- and postbronchodilator testing is frequently used to diagnose asthma. For this test, the individual completes a basic spirometry, followed by a bronchodilator. The spirometry is then repeated and evaluated for changes before and after the bronchodilator. The time interval between administration of the bronchodilator and the postbronchodilator testing varies. Data shows that the minimum interval should be 15–20 minutes for most short and intermediate-acting β_2 agonists.[5,6] An improvement in FEV_1 of >12% or an increase of ≥10% of predicted FEV_1 in response to bronchodilator treatment confirms reversible airway obstruction.

If the individual is a known asthmatic or has taken a bronchodilator within the last 4–6 hours, the test should be delayed to allow proper assessment of acute bronchodilator response. Long-acting inhaled bronchodilator use may require a longer delay in testing. For example salmeterol should be withheld for 12 hours, and ipratropium should be withheld for 6 hours. Medications taken on the day of testing, including OTC allergy formulas should be noted in the spirometry report.

Bronchoprovocation with methacholine is another test for asthma. Methacholine chloride is a synthetic choline ester that acts as a potent bronchoconstrictor. Most patients will return to their to baseline pulmonary function within 30–45 minutes of being challenged with methacholine or within 5 minutes of receiving an inhaled beta agonist. This study can also be conducted with inhaled histamine, adenosine, bradykinin, cold air, or exercise testing. The goal is to induce a bronchospasm. The format is essentially the same as a pre- and postbronchodilator test: basic spirometry is performed, the challenge is given, and then the spirometry is repeated so that the results can be compared. A decline in FEV_1 of 20% from baseline is considered a positive test for asthma. See Table 4.5 for definitions of some common pulmonary function tests (PFTs).

TABLE 4.5 Some Common Pulmonary Function Tests Used in Asthma Diagnosis

Measure	*Definition*	*What Does It Mean?*
FEV_1 (forced expiratory volume in 1 second)	Maximal volume forcibly exhaled within 1 second	• FEV_1 >80% of predicted = normal • FEV_1 60%–79% of predicted = mild obstruction • FEV_1 40%–59% of predicted = moderate obstruction • FEV_1 <40% of predicted = severe obstruction
FVC (forced vital capacity)	Total air forcibly exhaled after maximal inhalation	FVC is not a reliable indicator of total lung capacity or restriction, especially in the setting of airflow obstruction; however it can be an indicator of restrictive disease
FEV_1/FVC ratio	A calculated ratio of the proportion of the forced vital capacity exhaled in the first second	Ratio will be reduced in obstructive lung disease (COPD) and normal in restrictive lung disease (asthma)
FEF 25%–75%	Measures flow rates in the middle (25%—75%) of the FVC	Can reflect the function of the middle airways
Pre- and postbronchodilator testing	Basic spirometry, followed by a bronchodilator, and then spirometry is repeated to permit comparison	An improvement in FEV_1 of >12% or an increase ≥10% of predicted FEV_1 in response to bronchodilator treatment confirms reversible airway obstruction (asthma)
Maximum voluntary ventilation (MVV)	Maximum volume of air that can be exhaled over a specified period of time	Used to determine a person's breathing reserve Note: can trigger bronchospasm
Flow-volume loop	A graphic representation of maximal inhalation and exhalation	Measurement can indicate the location of airflow obstruction, such as the large upper airways or smaller distal airways
PEF (peak expiratory flow)	Fastest rate that air can be exhaled	Assesses expiratory muscle strength and large airway patency

(continues)

TABLE 4.5 Some Common Pulmonary Function Tests Used in Asthma Diagnosis *(Cont.)*

Measure	*Definition*	*What Does It Mean?*
Exhaled nitric oxide (NO)	Measurement of the percentage of exhaled nitric oxide	Can be a reflection of airway inflammation
DLCO (diffusing capacity of the lung for carbon monoxide)	Measurement of the partial pressure difference between inspired and expired carbon monoxide	Determines the ability of the lungs to transfer gases from the alveoli to the blood

Spirometry Complications and Contraindications

Spirometry is a useful diagnostic tool, but there are some complications and contraindications that practitioners should be aware of. Among these complications are: pneumothorax; increased intracranial pressure; dizziness, lightheadedness, or fainting; chest pain; coughing; bronchospasm; and oxygen desaturation due to the interruption of oxygen therapy. There are also instances when spirometry should be delayed until further evaluation of the individual's condition can be assessed. These are listed in Table 4.6.

TABLE 4.6 Contraindications for Spirometry

While spirometry can provide a window into lung function, there are times when spirometry should not be performed. Forced expiratory maneuvers may aggravate some medical conditions and should be postponed until the medical condition is resolved. Some of the conditions that may delay spirometry are:

- Hemoptysis of unknown origin
- Pneumothorax
- Unstable cardiovascular status (angina, recent myocardial infarction, etc.)
- Thoracic, abdominal, or cerebral aneurysms
- Cataracts or recent eye surgery
- Recent thoracic or abdominal surgery
- Nausea, vomiting, or acute illness
- Recent or current viral infection
- Young children who are unable to follow directions and/or safely complete the study

Adapted from: AARC Clinical Practice Guideline Spirometry, 1996 Update. http://www.rcjournal.com/cpgs/spirupdatecpg.html. Accessed May 22, 2009.[7]

Additional Testing

Once the initial assessment has been completed, additional testing may be required to further define the individual's pulmonary condition.

Allergy Testing

Determining the allergen responsible for triggering an asthmatic reaction can be very useful when developing control measures and limiting the individual's exposure. Provoking an allergic response, however, can be dangerous and should only be performed in a setting that can provide an emergency response. Among the types of skin tests approved for use in the United States are the prick test and the intracutaneous test. The prick test consists of pricking the skin with a needle that has been contaminated with the allergic antigen solution. The intracutaneous test involves injecting a small amount of the allergic antigen into the outer layers of the skin. This method is more accurate because the antigen is actually placed inside the body and the immune system can more fully respond. The skin patch test places the allergen solution on a pad that is taped to the individual's skin for 24–72 hours. This test is used most often to detect contact dermatitis. The Passive Transfer test is not used in the United States, however, it does still appear in some textbooks. This procedure includes the collection of test serum from an atopic individual, which is then injected intradermally into a normal/nonatopic subject. The normal subject is challenged 24–48 hours later with the antigen suspected of causing the immediate hypersensitivity reaction in the atopic individual to determine if there is hypersensitivity. The health risk of communicable diseases to the nonallergic test subject is considerable. This test is also known as a p-K test or Prausnitz-Küstner test. Dietary challenges include the omission of specific food believed to be causing a reaction. The food is added back to the diet, and the response is again gauged. This technique of allergen testing makes it difficult to quantify and measure the results. The antigen leukocyte cellular antibody test (ALCAT) is a blood test used for identification of foods, food additives, food colorings, and other chemicals that may cause hypersensitivities. It can be performed in a physician's office or at home with a special kit.

Biomarkers of Inflammation

In theory, the ability to measure the progression and occurrence of inflammation could be a good measure of asthma control. Studies are ongoing regarding the practical use of measuring biomarkers such as total and differential cell counts and mediator assays in asthmatics. The biomarkers can be found in sputum, blood, urine, and exhaled air. At this time there are no recommendations for their routine measurement in asthmatics.

Some Special Considerations

Data has shown that children 5 years of age and younger may have wheezing without having asthma. Children in this age group should be assessed carefully to determine their correct diagnosis and treatment options. Three categories of wheezing have been described in children 5 years and younger:

- Transient early wheezing that has been associated with prematurity and parental smoking. The children usually outgrow this by the age of 3 years. Parents should be encouraged not to smoke around their children.
- Persistent early-onset wheezing (before the age of 3 years) has been associated with acute viral respiratory infections. A clue that may be found in their medical history is that they have no atopy and no family history of atopy. Respiratory syncytial virus (RSV) in children younger than age 2 is usually the culprit and should be assessed. Other viruses appear to be the problem in older preschool children. Children with persistent early-onset wheezing may have symptoms throughout childhood that may still be present at 12 years of age.
- Late-onset wheezing/asthma. These children have asthma. They often also have symptoms of allergic atopy. They should be managed as asthmatics.[1]

Is It Asthma or COPD?

Both asthma and COPD involve underlying airway inflammation. In contrast to asthma, the inflammation associated with COPD is not triggered by allergen exposure and does not respond well to anti-inflammatory medication. COPD is characterized by airflow limitation that is not fully reversible and is usually progressive. With treatment, controlled asthma patients can have near-normal lung function and reversibility. The individual's history can also provide insights to the two conditions. A well-controlled asthmatic should not experience daily symptoms and should have near normal lung function. Individuals with COPD will not have normal PFTs and usually have symptoms daily.[8]

Referral to an Asthma Specialist for Consultation or Comanagement

Many asthmatic patients are managed by their family practice physician or their pediatrician. If their asthma is controlled and they are not in danger of a life-threatening exacerbation, this is safe and cost-effective. The current

U.S. guidelines recommend referral for consultation or care to a specialist in asthma if:

- The individual has had a life-threatening asthma exacerbation.
- The individual is not meeting the goals of asthma therapy after 3–6 months of treatment. An earlier referral or consultation is appropriate if the physician concludes that the individual is unresponsive to therapy.
- Signs and symptoms are atypical, or there are problems in differential diagnosis.
- Other conditions complicate asthma or its diagnosis (e.g., sinusitis, nasal polyps, aspergillosis, severe rhinitis, VCD, GERD, COPD).
- Additional diagnostic testing is indicated (e.g., allergy skin testing, rhinoscopy, complete pulmonary function studies, provocative challenge, bronchoscopy).
- The individual requires additional education and guidance on complications of therapy, problems with adherence, or allergen avoidance.
- The individual is being considered for immunotherapy.
- Referral is recommended if the individual requires Step 4 care or higher (Step 3 for children 0–4 years of age). Consider referral if the individual requires Step 3 care (Step 2 for children 0–4 years of age). (See Chapter 7 for the definitions of the steps used in asthma management.)
- The individual has required more than two bursts of oral corticosteroids in 1 year or has an exacerbation requiring hospitalization.
- The individual requires confirmation of a history that suggests that an occupational or environmental inhalant or ingested substance is provoking or contributing to asthma.

References

1. The Global Initiative for Asthma (GINA). 2009 Update of the GINA Report, Global Strategy for Asthma Management and Prevention. http://www.ginasthma.com/. Accessed April 1, 2010.
2. National Heart, Lung, and Blood Institute. National Asthma Education and Prevention Program Expert Panel Report 3: Guidelines for the Diagnosis and Management of Asthma Full Report 2007. http://www.nhlbi.nih.gov/guidelines/asthma/asthsumm.pdf. Accessed April 2, 2009.
3. Adams RJ, Smith BJ, Ruffin RE. Factors associated with hospital admissions and repeat emergency department visits for adults with asthma. *Thorax.* 2000;55(7):566–73.

4. Eisner MD, Katz PP, Yelin EH, Shiboski SC, Blanc PD. Risk factors for hospitalization among adults with asthma: the influence of sociodemographic factors and asthma severity. *Respir Res.* 2001;2(1):53–60.
5. Dales RE, Spitzer WO, Tousignant P, Schechter M, Suissa S. Clinical interpretation of airway response to bronchodilator: epidemiologic considerations. *Am Rev Respir Dis.* 1988;138(2):317–320.
6. Waalkens HJ, Merkus PJE, Essen-Zandvliet EEM, et al. Assessment of bronchodilator response in children with asthma. *Eur Respir J.* 1993;6:645–651.
7. AARC Clinical Practice Guideline Spirometry, 1996 Update. http://www.rcjournal.com/cpgs/spirupdatecpg.html. Accessed May 22, 2009.
8. Smart BA. When Asthma and COPD Coexist. American Academy of Allergy, Asthma, and Immunology. June 2007. http://www.aaaai.org/patients/seniorsandasthma/when_asthma_copd_coexist.stm. Accessed June 12, 2009.

5

Asthma Severity

LEARNING OBJECTIVES

- Review the goals of asthma therapy
- Discuss the classifications of asthma severity
- Define the term asthma control
- Identify strategies and techniques for ongoing asthma monitoring

KEY WORDS

intermittent asthma
mild persistent asthma
moderate persistent asthma
severe persistent asthma
asthma control
stepwise therapy
stepdown therapy
asthma control plan
patient diary

Introduction

Once the diagnosis of asthma has been established, determining the appropriate treatment level is essential to safely and effectively manage the individual's condition. Traditionally, practitioners have classified an individual's asthma by its severity as intermittent, mild persistent, moderate persistent, and severe persistent. These classifications have been used to guide the necessary levels of treatment. The revised 2009 GINA guidelines, however, now recommend that this classification by severity be used for research purposes only. The GINA guidelines recommend using levels of control as a guide to determine appropriate treatment decisions. The GINA-recommended levels of control are: controlled, partly controlled, or uncontrolled asthma. The rationale behind using these categories is that they include a measure of the severity of the underlying disease and also the current state of responsiveness to treatment.

The achievement of control and maintaining asthma control are goals of the current U.S. guidelines; however, the classification system and recommendations are still based on measures of severity. Regardless of which classification system is used, treatment options should be clearly spelled out in a written asthma action plan that can alert the individual when his or her asthma is deteriorating. The asthma action plan can not only help identify an impeding exacerbation, but provide individuals with the tools they need to prevent their condition from worsening and alert them when they need to seek assistance.

Classifying Asthma by Severity

Asthma severity can be classified based on the level of symptoms individuals are experiencing, their degree of airflow limitation, and their lung function variability. Using these measures, asthma can be divided into four categories of severity. They are: intermittent, mild persistent, moderate persistent, or severe persistent. The U.S. guidelines make specific recommendations per age group for each of these classifications of severity.[1] The age groups are: 0–4 years of age; children 5–11 years of age; and youth ≥ 12 years of age and adults. The following chapters will address the specific recommendations for these age groups in greater detail.

Classifying Asthma by Control

The 2009 GINA guidelines classify asthma as controlled, partly controlled, and uncontrolled. They stress that the goal of treatment should be to achieve and maintain control for prolonged periods of time. Table 5.1 lists the GINA-recommended definition levels of asthma control.

Goals of Asthma Control

Both the U.S. and the international guidelines stress the importance of gaining control of asthma. They define control as not only managing symptoms, but also reducing inflammation and minimizing long-term disease progression. The specific goals of asthma control are reducing impairment

TABLE 5.1 Levels of Asthma Control

Controlled Asthma

- Daytime symptoms: Twice or less per week
- Limitations of activities: None
- Nocturnal symptoms/awakening: None
- Need for reliever/rescue treatment: Twice or less per week
- Lung function (PEF or FEV_1): Normal

Partly Controlled Asthma

- Daytime symptoms: More than twice per week
- Limitations of activities: Any
- Nocturnal symptoms/awakening: Any
- Need for reliever/rescue treatment: More than twice per week
- Lung function (PEF or FEV_1): < 80% predicted or personal best (lung function is not a reliable test for children 5 years and younger)

Uncontrolled Asthma

- Three or more features of partly controlled asthma present in any week
- The occurrence of an exacerbation should be considered as a symptom of uncontrolled asthma and requires further evaluation of asthma status.

Adapted from: The Global Initiative for Asthma (GINA). 2009 Update of the GINA Report, Global Strategy for Asthma Management and Prevention. http://www.ginasthma.com. Accessed April 12, 2010.

and minimizing the risk of recurrent exacerbations and progressive loss of lung function (see Table 5.2). From a clinical perspective, this translates as individuals' asthma being controlled if they experience little or no clinical symptoms and have a near normal pulmonary function study.

Asthma is determined to be controlled if the individual experiences little or no clinical symptoms and has a near normal pulmonary function study.

Both the U.S. and the international guidelines recommend using a stepwise approach to pharmacologic therapy to gain and maintain control of asthma and reduce both impairment and risk of exacerbations and progression. Once control of the individual's asthma is established, stepdown therapy should be considered, so as to use the minimum amount of medication necessary to maintain control. Monitoring asthma becomes essential to regulating this stepwise approach (either up or down) for asthma.

TABLE 5.2 The Goals of Asthma Control

Reducing impairment	Prevent chronic and troublesome symptoms (e.g., coughing or breathlessness during daytime, in the night, or after exertion)
	Require infrequent use (≤ 2 days a week) of inhaled short-acting beta$_2$-agonist (SABA) for quick relief of symptoms (not including prevention of exercise-induced bronchospasm [EIB])
	Maintain (near) normal pulmonary function
	Maintain normal activity levels (including exercise and other physical activity, and attendance at work or school)
	Meet individuals' and families' expectations of, and satisfaction with, asthma treatment
Reducing risk	Prevent recurrent exacerbations of asthma and minimize the need for emergency department (ED) visits or hospitalizations
	Prevent progressive loss of lung function; for children, prevent reduced lung growth
	Provide optimal pharmacotherapy with minimal or no adverse effects

Adapted from: National Heart, Lung, and Blood Institute. National Asthma Education and Prevention Program Expert Panel Report 3: Guidelines for the Diagnosis and Management of Asthma Full Report 2007. http://www.nhlbi.nih.gov/guidelines/asthma/asthsumm.pdf. Accessed April 2, 2009.

Monitoring Asthma

Monitoring asthma is essential to gaining and maintaining control. A basic asthma monitoring program should be a joint effort between the health-care provider and the individual. Regular follow-up visits should assess the following:

- Signs and symptoms of asthma
- Pulmonary function status (spirometry; peak flow monitoring)
- Quality of life
- Recent history of asthma exacerbations
- Pharmacotherapy adherence and any potential side effects
- Satisfaction with their asthma management plan

The plan may also include measurement of minimally invasive markers and pharmacogenetics where possible.[1]

Monitoring Signs and Symptoms of Asthma

Measuring the signs and symptoms of asthma can provide a direct window into how the patient is in need of intervention, or if the current plan is adequately controlling their asthma. One of the best ways to assess signs and symptoms is through the review of the individual's symptom diary. This is simply a daily log of whether or not they are experiencing symptoms and may include their daily peak flow measurement readings. A consistently kept diary can reveal trends in asthma severity and help identify potential triggers of the individual's asthma symptoms.

Peak Flow Monitoring

Daily monitoring of the individual's peak flow rate is a useful tool for assessing asthma control and can be easily incorporated into the asthma diary. Incorporating the peak flow zone system into their plan helps to quantify the individual's level of control. To use the zone system, the individual's asthma ideally should be controlled. They should monitor their peak flows daily for a 2- to 3-week period. Their personal best is the highest number achieved during this time. This number is then used as the basis for the peak flow zone system. The system uses three color-coded ranges signifying the individual's personal best peak flow measurements. The green zone is defined as 80%–100% of their personal best peak flow range, the yellow zone is defined as 50%–80% of their personal best, and the red zone is defined as below 50% of their personal best. Table 5.3 illustrates a sample patient diary that incorporates the zone system.

The individuals' diary and symptoms should be assessed at each follow-up visit to determine if their asthma is controlled or if a change in their plan is necessary.

Monitoring Pulmonary Function Status

Assessment of the individual's pulmonary function status, including peak flow measurement and spirometry, should be done regularly. Ongoing daily peak flow monitoring should be considered in individuals who:

- have moderate or severe persistent asthma.
- have a history of severe exacerbations.
- have poorly perceived airflow obstruction and worsening asthma.
- prefer this type of monitoring over a symptom-based monitoring plan.

Spirometry should be performed upon initial assessment, once asthma control is attained, and to document (near) normal lung function. Spirometry should also be performed in the event of a progressive or prolonged loss of

TABLE 5.3 Daily Asthma Monitoring

My **green zone** peak flow is above: __________. My symptoms are: no coughing or wheezing; I slept through the night; I can work/play without difficulty.

My yellow zone peak flow is between: _________ and ________. My symptoms are: I am getting a cold/infection; I have been exposed to a known trigger/allergen; I am coughing; I am wheezing; I have tightness in my chest; my asthma woke me up last night.

(Caution: see asthma action plan.)

My red zone peak flow is below: __________. My symptoms are: my rescue medicine is not helping within 15–20 minutes; I am wheezing and/or my breathing is hard and fast; my lips and/or fingernails are blue; I am having difficulty walking and/or talking.

(Danger: see asthma action plan immediately!)

Date/time	*Morning PEF*	*Evening PEF*	*My symptoms today are:*	*Rescue medication used: (time and number of puffs)*	*Symptoms relieved (yes/no/ time)*
Monday					
Tuesday					
Wednesday					
Thursday					
Friday					
Saturday					
Sunday					
Quality of life/ satisfaction Assessment	This week I missed ________ day(s) of work/school. I was/was not able to participate in home/work/school/recreation/ exercise. My asthma directly impacted my: mom/dad/spouse/other. My asthma plan worked/did not work for me this week. My plan would be better if:				

asthma control and at least every 1–2 years to monitor any changes that may be occurring in the airway.[1]

Symptom-based monitoring plans work on the same principle as the peak flow plan. They incorporate a zone system that identifies when action should be taken to halt an asthma attack. The plan incorporates both a symptom and a peak flow daily monitoring system. Table 5.4 illustrates a standalone symptom monitoring system.

TABLE 5.4 Daily Asthma Symptom Monitoring

In my **green zone** my symptoms are: no coughing or wheezing; I slept through the night; I can work/play without difficulty.

In my **yellow zone** my symptoms are: I am getting a cold/infection; I have been exposed to a known trigger/allergen; I am coughing; I am wheezing; I have tightness in my chest; my asthma woke me up last night.

(Caution: see asthma action plan.)

In my **red zone** my symptoms are: my rescue medicine is not helping within 15–20 minutes; I am wheezing and/or my breathing is hard and fast; my lips and/or fingernails are blue; I am having difficulty walking and/or talking.

(Danger: see asthma action plan immediately!)

Date/time	*Symptoms I am experiencing:*	*Rescue medication used: (time and number of puffs)*	*Symptoms relieved: (yes/no/time)*
Monday			
Tuesday			
Wednesday			
Thursday			
Friday			
Saturday			
Sunday			
Quality of life/ satisfaction assessment	This week I missed _______ day(s) of work/school. I was/was not able to participate in home/work/school/ recreation/exercise. My asthma directly impacted my: mom/dad/spouse/other. My asthma plan worked/did not work for me this week. My plan would be better if:		

Monitoring Quality of Life

Monitoring for changes in the individual's quality of life and any impact on their school/work performance is critical and should be assessed during each visit. The preceding sample diaries provide for this quality of life assessment.

Monitoring History of Asthma Exacerbations

Documenting the severity and frequency of an exacerbation should be completed at every office visit. Monitoring these parameters can help to guide stepwise therapy and identify periods when the individual is particularly vulnerable to triggers. For example, if it is documented that pollen in the springtime triggers exacerbations in individuals, adjustment in their medication can be made to prevent worsening of their asthma during this season.

Monitoring Pharmacotherapy Adherence and Side Effects

At each visit the individual's adherence to their medication plan, inhaler technique, and any potential side effects that they maybe having should be assessed. This is also a good time to discuss their overall satisfaction with their asthma action plan and confirm that there is effective communication between individuals and their providers. Effective, open communication is essential to providing quality care and any concerns should be addressed. A frequently heard concern is that individuals are not sure who they should call in the event of an emergency or if they have questions about their medications. Resolving these issues can facilitate better care and prevent them from unnecessary emergency and office visits.

Follow-Up Checklist

A sample checklist for a follow-up visit, which covers all of these areas, is illustrated in Table 5.5.

TABLE 5.5 Sample Routine Clinical Assessment Questionnaire*

Question	*Individual's Response*	*Action to Be Taken*
Monitoring signs and symptoms		
"Has your asthma been better or worse since your last visit?"		
"Has your asthma worsened during specific seasons or events?"		
"In the past 2 weeks, how many days have you:		
• Had problems with coughing, wheezing, shortness of breath, or chest tightness during the day?"		
• Awakened at night from sleep because of coughing or other asthma symptoms?"		
• Awakened in the morning with asthma symptoms that did not improve within 15 minutes of inhaling a short-acting $beta_2$-agonist?"		
• Had symptoms while exercising or playing?"		
• Been unable to perform a usual activity, including exercise, because of asthma?"		
Monitoring pulmonary functions		
Lung function		
"What is the highest and lowest your peak flow has been since your last visit?"		
"Has your peak flow dropped below ___ L/min (80% of personal best) since your last visit?" "What did you do when this occurred?"		
Peak flow monitoring technique		
"Please show me how you measure your peak flow." "When do you usually measure your peak flow?"		

(continues)

TABLE 5.5 Sample Routine Clinical Assessment Questionnaire *(Cont.)*

Question	*Individual's Response*	*Action to Be Taken*
Monitoring quality of life/functional status		
"Since your last visit, how many days has your asthma caused you to:		
• miss work or school?"		
• reduce your activities?"		
• (for caregivers) change your activity because of your child's asthma?"		
"Since your last visit, have you had any unscheduled or emergency department visits or hospital stays?"		
Monitoring exacerbation history		
Since your last visit, have you had any episodes/ times when your asthma symptoms were much worse than usual?" **If yes**, "What do you think caused the symptoms to get worse?" **If yes**, "What did you do to control the symptoms?"		
"Have there been any changes in your home or work environment (e.g., new smokers or pets)?"		
Monitoring pharmacotherapy		
Medications		
"What medications are you taking?"		
"How do you feel about taking medication?"		
"How often do you take each medication?"		
"How much do you take each time?"		
"Have you missed or stopped taking any regular doses of your medications for any reason?" **If yes**, why?		
"Have you had trouble filling your prescriptions (e.g., for financial reasons, not on formulary)?"		

TABLE 5.5 Sample Routine Clinical Assessment Questionnaire *(Cont.)*

Question	*Individual's Response*	*Action to Be Taken*
"How many puffs of your inhaled short-acting beta$_2$-agonist (quick-relief medicine) do you use per day?"		
"How many [name inhaled short-acting beta$_2$-agonist] inhalers [or pumps] have you been through in the past month?"		
"Have you tried any other medicines or remedies?"		
Side effects		
"Has your asthma medicine caused you any problems?"		
(shakiness, nervousness, bad taste, sore throat, cough, upset stomach, hoarseness, skin changes [e.g., bruising])		
Inhaler technique		
"Please show me how you use your inhaler."		
Monitoring patient–provider communication and patient satisfaction		
"What questions have you had about your asthma daily self-management plan and action plan?"		
"What problems have you had following your daily self-management plan? Your action plan?"		
"How do you feel about making your own decisions about therapy?"		
"Has anything prevented you from getting the treatment you need for your asthma from me or anyone else?"		
"Have the costs of your asthma treatment interfered with your ability to get asthma care?"		
"How satisfied are you with your asthma care?"		
"How can we improve your asthma care?"		
"Let's review some important information:		
• When should you increase your medications? Which medication(s)?"		

(continues)

TABLE 5.5 Sample Routine Clinical Assessment Questionnaire *(Cont.)*

Question	*Individual's Response*	*Action to Be Taken*
• When should you call me [your doctor or nurse practitioner]? Do you know the after-hours phone number?"		
• If you can't reach me/this clinic, what emergency department would you go to?"		

*These questions are examples and do not represent a standardized assessment instrument. The validity and reliability of these questions have not been assessed.

Adapted from: National Heart, Lung, and Blood Institute. National Asthma Education and Prevention Program Expert Panel Report 3: Guidelines for the Diagnosis and Management of Asthma Full Report 2007. http://www.nhlbi.nih.gov/guidelines/asthma/asthsumm.pdf. Accessed April 2, 2009.

Recommended Monitoring/Visit Schedules

The scheduling and the frequency of follow-up visits to review asthma control are a matter of clinical judgment. Table 5.6 illustrates some recommended schedules.

TABLE 5.6 Recommended Monitoring Schedules

When starting therapy	2- to 6-week intervals until asthma control is achieved
Regular follow-up	Individuals who have intermittent or mild persistent asthma that has been under control for at least 3 months should be seen by a clinician about every 6 months.
	Individuals who have uncontrolled and/or severe persistent asthma and those who need additional supervision to help them follow their treatment plan need to be seen more often.
If a step down in therapy is anticipated	Consider 3-month intervals for monitoring

Adapted from: The Global Initiative for Asthma. 2009 Update of the GINA Report, Global Strategy for Asthma Management and Prevention. http://www.ginasthma.com. Accessed April 1, 2010.[2]

National Heart, Lung, and Blood Institute. National Asthma Education and Prevention Program Expert Panel Report 3: Guidelines for the Diagnosis and Management of Asthma Full Report 2007. http://www.nhlbi.nih.gov/guidelines/asthma/asthsumm.pdf. Accessed April 2, 2009.[1]

References

1. National Heart, Lung, and Blood Institute. National Asthma Education and Prevention Program Expert Panel Report 3: Guidelines for the Diagnosis and Management of Asthma Full Report 2007. http://www.nhlbi.nih.gov/guidelines/asthma/asthsumm.pdf. Accessed April 2, 2009.
2. The Global Initiative for Asthma (GINA). 2009 Update of the GINA Report, Global Strategy for Asthma Management and Prevention. http://www.ginasthma.com. Accessed April 1, 2010.

6 Medications

LEARNING OBJECTIVES

- Review the proper use of a spacer device with adults and children
- Discuss the use of reliever medication for wheezing and other acute symptoms
- Discuss the use of long-term controllers for the management of asthma

KEY WORDS

short-acting beta agonists (SABAs)
systemic corticosteroids
anticholinergic medications
spacer devices
methylxanthines
mast cell inhibitors
immunomodulators
long-acting beta agonists (LABAs)
leukotriene modifiers
inhaled corticosteroids
leukotriene modifiers
cromolyn

Introduction

The goals of asthma therapy are to gain control, reduce impairment and the risk of exacerbations, minimize side effects from medications, and maintain pulmonary function studies as close to normal as possible. Medications for asthma are categorized into two general classes: quick-relief medications used to treat acute symptoms and exacerbations and long-term control medications used to achieve and maintain control of persistent asthma. Systemic corticosteroids are usually considered long-term control when they are used to facilitate recovery from an exacerbation.

Quick-Relief Medications

Short-Acting Beta Agonists

Quick-relief medications, also called reliever medications or rescue medications, are used to provide relief of wheezing (bronchoconstriction) and other acute symptoms such as cough and tightness in the chest. Short-acting beta agonists (SABAs) and anticholinergics (ipratropium bromide) are the two principal reliever medications available in the United States.[1]

The SABAs relax smooth muscle and restore/increase airflow usually within 3–5 minutes of proper administration. These medications interact with beta to relax bronchial smooth muscle; decrease mast cell mediator release; and inhibit neutrophil, eosinophil, and lymphocyte functional responses. They also increase mucociliary transport and affect vascular tone and edema formation. SABAs are the therapy of choice for relief of acute asthma symptoms. Daily routine use of SABAs is not recommended and the use of these medications more than 2 days a week for symptom relief is considered an indicator of poorly controlled asthma.

SABAs are also the medication of choice for the prevention of exercise-induced asthma. For this indication it should be used before exercise and the caution against using these medications more than 2 days a week does not apply.[1] When SABAs are not tolerated, anticholinergics (ipratropium bromide) are the recommended alternative.

Short-Acting Beta Agonists Available in the United States

Albuterol (Ventolin, Proventil)

Levalbuterol (Xopenex)

Metaproterenol (Alupent, Metaprel)

Pirbuterol (Maxair)

The preferred delivery method for SABAs is inhalation. The medication itself can be formulated either in a metered-dose inhaler (MDI), breath-activated inhaler, or dry-powder inhaler (DPI) or administered via a nebulizer. Data has shown that delivery via an inhaler plus a spacer is as effective as nebulizer therapy when proper technique is used.[2] The recommended delivery method for children younger than 4 years of age is a pressurized metered dose inhaler used with a spacer device and a face mask. Children 4–6 years of age should use a pressurized metered-dose inhaler with a spacer device and a mouthpiece. Children and adults older than 6 years of age may use a dry powder inhaler, breath-actuated pressurized metered dose inhaler, or pressurized metered-dose inhaler with a spacer device and mouthpiece. A valved spacer device or holding chamber can also be used for adults and older children. Valved holding chambers (VHC) are essentially spacer devices that have one-way valves that do not allow exhalation into the device. This is beneficial for young children, infants, and those who are unable to coordinate their breathing. They can breathe normally and have someone else actuate the device without loss of the actuated dose of medication. Nebulizer therapy is an alternative regardless of the age group. However, children less than 4 years of age should use a mask with their nebulizer; all others may use a mouthpiece.[3] Oral administration of SABAs results in a slower onset of action and is not the preferred delivery route to quickly relieve symptoms.[1]

How to Use a Spacer Device

1. Sit or stand up as straight as possible, and take several deep breaths.
2. Remove the cap from the mouthpiece of the inhaler and shake the inhaler before use (3–4 shakes).
3. Some medications require "priming" or activating the inhaler prior to using. Please check to see if your inhaler requires this.
4. Insert the inhaler mouthpiece into the spacer device.
5. Place the spacer device in your mouth and seal your lips tightly around the spacer mouthpiece.
6. With the spacer still in your mouth, press down on the inhaler canister to spray one puff of medicine into the spacer.
7. Breathe in slowly and deeply through the spacer and hold your breath for 10 seconds or as long as is comfortably possible.
8. If the medication plan calls for 2 puffs of medication, wait 30–60 seconds, shake the inhaler again then repeat Steps 3–7.

Using a Spacer Device Fitted with a Mask for a Small Child

1. Place the child on your lap. Preferably with the child's head against your chest for support.
2. Remove the cap from the mouthpiece of the inhaler and shake the inhaler before use (3–4 shakes; prime inhaler if necessary).

3. Insert the inhaler mouthpiece into the spacer device.
4. Place the mask over the child's face so that the nose and mouth are covered.
5. Spray one puff from the inhaler into the spacer device.
6. Keep the mask in place for 6–8 breaths.
7. Have the child hold his/her breath, if possible, for a count of 10.
8. Remove the mask and repeat if necessary.

How to Clean a Spacer Device

1. Take the spacer device apart.
2. Swish the parts of the spacer device in warm soapy water (dish detergent works well).
3. Do not use boiling water, alcohol, bleach, or other cleaners or disinfectants as this may damage the spacer device.
4. Rinse well in clean water.
5. Let air dry.
6. Put the spacer back together.

Anticholinergics

Anticholinergic medications (ipratropium bromide) decrease bronchospasm and the secretion of mucus by inhibiting the muscarinic cholinergic receptors and reducing the vagal tone of the airway. They have an additive benefit when administered with SABAs in moderate to severe asthma exacerbations.

Anticholinergic Medication Available in the United States

Ipratropium bromide (Atrovent)

Systemic Corticosteroids

Systemic corticosteroids are neither rapid nor short acting. They are sometimes included in a reliever plan; usually in cases of moderate and severe exacerbations. These corticosteroids speed recovery from airway inflammation and hopefully prevent recurrence of another acute exacerbation. They can be given via injections, intravenously (IV), or orally. Most often the use of a short course (e.g., 3 days) of oral corticosteroids is seen following a moderate or severe exacerbation.

Long-Term Control Medications

Corticosteroids

Corticosteroids are the most potent and effective anti-inflammatory medications currently available and as such are used as controller medications for asthma. The current U.S. guidelines recommend their use as long-term therapy for mild, moderate, or severe persistent asthma. They state that, in general, these medications are well tolerated and safe at the recommended dosages. Oral and intravenous corticosteroids may be given in an emergency to gain control of an asthma exacerbation or as a bridge to inhaled therapy following a severe exacerbation. The preferred method of delivery, however, is via inhalation as this will deliver the medication locally to the pulmonary tissue where it is most needed, reduce the degree of systemic exposure, and decrease the risk of side effects. The risk of adverse effects from corticosteroids increases with higher dose and potency levels. To minimize these risks practitioners should recommend the lowest dose possible to maintain asthma control. Patients can also decrease their side effects when taking inhaled corticosteroids (ICS) by using a spacer device with good technique and rinsing their mouths afterward to remove any residue. The guidelines and data suggest that there is a small risk of adverse events from the use of ICS, but that their efficacy balances this risk (see Table 6.1).[1]

More details regarding dosing and the use of corticosteroids addressing specific age groups are discussed in the following chapters. Regardless of the age of the individual, corticosteroids should not be used to relieve symptoms during an acute asthma attack!

TABLE 6.1 Adverse Effects from Inhaled Corticosteroids

Local adverse effects	Oropharyngeal candidiasis Dysphonia (difficulty speaking) Occasional coughing from upper airway irritation
Systemic side effects of long-term treatment with high doses of inhaled corticosteroids	Easy bruising Adrenal suppression Decreased bone mineral density (BMD)

TABLE 6.1 Adverse Effects from Inhaled Corticosteroids (*Cont.*)

Specific Situations	
Cataracts	Inhaled corticosteroids have been associated with the occurrence of cataracts and glaucoma. There is no evidence of posterior-subcapsular cataracts.
Bone density	Calcium (1000–1500 mg per day) and vitamin D (400–800 units per day) supplements should be considered for patients who have risk factors for osteoporosis or low bone mineral density. Bone-sparing therapy (e.g., bisphosphonate) may be considered for patients on medium or high doses of ICS, particularly for those who are at risk of osteoporosis or who have low BMD scores by dual energy X-ray absorptiometry (or DEXA) scan. For children, age-appropriate dietary intake of calcium and exercise should be reviewed with the child's caregivers.
Pulmonary infections	There is no evidence that the use of ICS increases the risk of pulmonary infections, including tuberculosis.

Adapted from: The Global Initiative for Asthma (GINA). 2009 Update of the GINA Report, Global Strategy for Asthma Management and Prevention. http://www.ginasthma.com. Accessed April 1, 2010.[4]

Corticosteroids Available in the United States

Oral and Intravenous Corticosteroids

Methylprednisolone (Medrol, Solu-Medrol)

Prednisone (Deltasone, Orasone)

Prednisolone (Pediapred, Orapred)

Inhaled Corticosteroids

Beclomethasone (Beclovent, Vanceril, Qvar)

Budesonide (Pulmicort)

Flunisolide (AeroBid)

Fluticasone (Flovent)

Triamcinolone (Azmacort)

Mast Cell Inhibitors

Cromolyn sodium and nedocromil are anti-inflammatory medications that stabilize mast cells and interfere with chloride channel function. The current U.S. guidelines state that they may be used as an alternative, but are not the preferred medications for the treatment of mild persistent asthma. They can also be used as preventive treatment before exercise or unavoidable exposure to known allergens. The data shows that while both medications are potent anti-inflammatory agents, nedocromil may be more potent than cromolyn in inhibiting bronchospasm provoked by exercise.

Mast Cell Inhibitors Available in the United States

Cromolyn sodium (Intal)

Nedocromil (Tilade)

Immunomodulators

Currently the only immunomodulator available in the United States is the monoclonal antibody omalizumab (anti-IgE). Omalizumab prevents binding of IgE to the high-affinity receptors on basophils and mast cells, thus interrupting and decreasing the release of mediators in response to allergen exposure. It is recommended for the long-term control and prevention of symptoms for patients older than 12 years of age that have moderate or severe persistent allergic asthma inadequately controlled with ICS. Clinicians who administer omalizumab are cautioned that they should be prepared and equipped to identify and treat anaphylaxis should it occur.

Monoclonal Antibodies Available in the United States

Omalizumab (Xolair)

Leukotriene Modifiers

Three leukotriene modifiers—montelukast, zafirlukast, and zileuton—are available as oral tablets for the treatment of asthma. These are further divided into two pharmacologic classes: 5-lipoxygenase pathway inhibitors (e.g., zileuton) and receptor antagonists (LTRAs; montelukast and zafirlukast), which block the effects of the CysLT1 receptor. The current U.S. guidelines recommend that LTRAs be used as an alternative treatment option for mild persistent asthma. They can also be used as adjunct therapy with

ICS. In patients 12 years of age and older they are not the preferred adjunct therapy compared to the addition of long-acting beta agonists (LABAs). The 5-lipoxygenase pathway inhibitor zileuton is an alternative treatment option, though the guidelines state its use is less desirable than LTRAs due to more limited efficacy data and the need for liver function monitoring.[1]

Leukotriene Modifiers Available in the United States

Leukotriene receptor antagonists (LTRAs)	Montelukast (Singulair) Zafirlukast (Accolate)
5-Lipoxygenase pathway inhibitors	Zileuton (Zyflo)

Long-Acting Beta Agonists

There are two long acting beta agonists (LABAs) available in the United States: salmeterol and formoterol. These medications are bronchodilators that have an efficacy lasting up to 12 hours; they are not, however, to be used as monotherapy for long-term control of asthma. These medications are most often used in combination with ICS for long-term control and prevention of symptoms. LABAs should not be used for the treatment of acute symptoms or exacerbations. There has been some controversy regarding whether or not LABA treatment increases the severity of asthma exacerbations and possibly increases the risk of mortality. Data from the Salmeterol Multi-center Asthma Research Trial (SMART), a large 28-week, placebo-controlled U.S. study that examined the safety of salmeterol added to usual asthma therapy, demonstrated that individuals taking salmeterol showed a small but significant increase in asthma-related deaths (13 deaths out of 13,176 patients) compared to those individuals on placebo therapy (3 out of 13,179). These concerns have resulted in a black box warning from the FDA on LABAs and ICS combination products. Individuals using LABAs should be instructed not to stop their ICS therapy while taking these medications.[1,5,6]

Long-Acting Beta Agonists (LABAs) Available in the United States

Formoterol (Foradil)

Salmeterol (Serevent)

Combined Controller Therapy

There are two combined products currently available in the United States for the long-term control of asthma. These products include an inhaled corticosteroid and a LABA. The combinations currently available are: fluticasone and salmeterol (Advair) and budesonide and formoterol (Symbicort). These medications should be used as controller therapy and not in place of rescue medications.

Methylxanthines

Methylxanthines provide mild-to-moderate relaxation of airway smooth muscles and help to decrease the occurrence of bronchospasms. Similar to caffeine, these medications are nonselective phosphodiesterase inhibitors that also have a mild anti-inflammatory effect. The methylxanthine most commonly used in the United States is theophylline. The current guidelines recommend that sustained-release theophylline be used as an alternative rather than a preferred treatment for mild persistent asthma. It may also be used as alternative but not preferred adjunctive therapy with ICS. Too much theophylline can result in toxicity, which is most often represented as severe headaches, tachycardia, tremors, muscle twitching, seizures, nausea, and vomiting. To prevent these side effects and insure a therapeutic range, monitoring of serum concentrations of theophylline should be done. When using sustained-release theophyllines, serum concentration levels should be obtained in the middle of the dosing interval, at least 3–5 days after initiation of therapy. Serum levels should also be obtained at least 2 days after initiation of any factor known to affect theophylline clearance significantly such as alterations in kidney function, sepsis, thyroid disease, pregnancy, liver disease, and smoking. The therapeutic range for serum theophylline levels is 5–20 mcg/mL. Usually maintaining peak serum theophylline levels between 10 and 15 mcg/mL will achieve most of the drug's potential therapeutic benefit, however individuals with mild asthma may require lower levels. Serum theophylline levels > 20 mcg/mL increase both the frequency and severity of adverse reactions increase. Data has also been shown that theophylline clearance is increased and half-life decreased by low carbohydrate/high protein diets, parenteral nutrition, and daily consumption of charcoal-broiled beef. A high carbohydrate/low protein diet can decrease the clearance and prolong the half-life of theophylline.[7]

References

1. National Heart, Lung, and Blood Institute. National Asthma Education and Prevention Program Expert Panel Report 3: Guidelines for the Diagnosis and Management of Asthma Full Report 2007. http://www.nhlbi.nih.gov/guidelines/asthma/asthsumm.pdf. Accessed April 2, 2009.

2. Dhuper S, Chandra A, Ahmed A. Efficacy and cost comparisons of bronchodilator administration between metered dose inhalers with disposable spacers and nebulizers for acute asthma in an inner-city adult population. *J Emerg Med*. December 10, 2008. [Epub ahead of print.]
3. Newman KB, Milne S, Hamilton C, Hall K. A comparison of albuterol administered by metered-dose inhaler and spacer with albuterol by nebulizer in adults presenting to an urban emergency department with acute asthma. *Chest*. 2002;121(4):1036–41.
4. The Global Initiative for Asthma (GINA). 2009 Update of the GINA Report, Global Strategy for Asthma Management and Prevention. http://www.ginasthma.com. Accessed April 1, 2010.
5. American Academy of Pediatrics. FDA adds black box warning to long-acting beta agonists. *AAP News*. 2006;27(2):27. http://www.aap.org/sections/socpt/27.pdf. Accessed December 26, 2009.
6. Nelson HS, Weiss ST, Bleecker ER, et al. Salmeterol Multi-Center Asthma Research Trial (SMART). *Chest*. 2006;129(1):15–26.
7. Package insert for Theophylline. http://www.frx.com/pi/Theophylline_pi.pdf. Accessed July 26, 2009.

7 Stepwise Management, Asthma Action Plans, and Patient Education

LEARNING OBJECTIVES

- Discuss stepwise management for the control of asthma
- Review the components of an asthma action plan
- Discuss the use of a school/sports action plan
- Identify the components of a patient education plan
- Discuss the development of a patient/provider partnership

KEY WORDS

stepwise management
asthma action plan
school/sports action plan
travel plan
green zone
yellow zone
red zone

Introduction

Both U.S. and international guidelines recommend using a stepwise approach to pharmacologic therapy to gain and maintain control of asthma and reduce both impairment and risk of exacerbations and progression.[1,2] Written asthma action plans not only help individuals track and implement the stepwise approach, it allows asthmatics to daily monitor and adjust their medications in response to changing signs and symptoms thus reducing their risk of exacerbations. Every asthmatic should have a written asthma action plan.

Stepwise Management

The stepwise management plan organizes asthma treatment into different steps or levels based on the individual's signs and symptoms at that moment and reflects increasing and decreasing intensity of treatment (dosages and/or number of medications) required to achieve and maintain asthma control. The steps are determined on a case-by-case basis with respect to the age of the individual and severity of their asthma. The medication, dosage, and timing of the therapy are determined by the level of asthma severity assessed at the initiation of therapy and the level of asthma control needed for adjusting therapy. By utilizing the stepwise management plan, therapy can be stepped up or down as needed to maintain control. The goal for step-down therapy is to identify the minimum medication necessary to maintain control. Detailed information on stepwise management by age group and in accordance with the current U.S. guidelines is included in the following chapters.

Asthma Action Plan

A written asthma action plan is a document developed jointly by the health-care provider and the individual. The plan should include individuals' daily treatment plans, key points to help them recognize changes in their condition, and steps they can take to manage these changes. The patients' ability to self-adjust their medications in response to acute symptoms or changes in their PEF measurements is the basis of most written plans.

An asthma action plan should include two sections as a minimum: daily management and emergency response. The daily management section should incorporate directions for the daily management of their asthma including the names of the medications, dosages, and times they should be taken. It should also include daily monitoring information, steps to control environmental allergens, and directions for avoiding any known triggers.

The emergency response section should include information on how to recognize symptom changes and the specific steps (i.e., medications to take, dosage, and timing) they should follow in response to these changes. It is critical that the plan include information on the identification of signs, symptoms, and PEF measurements that indicate the need for urgent medical attention. Individuals with asthma and their immediate care providers must be provided with the red zone parameters that indicate the need for professional care beyond this point. It is a good idea that the written asthma plan also include emergency telephone numbers for the physician, nearest emergency department, and any emergency transport system/service that individuals can call quickly to assist them. See Table 7.1 for a sample of a written asthma action plan.

TABLE 7.1 Sample Asthma Action Plan

Name:	Address:		In case of an emergency please contact:	
Allergies/known triggers:			Physician/clinic Emergency contact:	
Short-acting reliever medications for asthma:				
Medication:			Dosage:	
Controller medications for asthma:				
Medication:			Dosage:	
Other medications I am taking:				
Green Zone No coughing or wheezing I slept through the night I can work/play without difficulty	80%–100% of my personal best My peak flow is above _______	Action to be taken when in the green zone:	Time action taken:	Did it help?

Yellow Zone I am getting a cold/infection I have been exposed to a known trigger/allergen I am coughing I am wheezing I have tightness in my chest My asthma woke me up last night	50%–80% of my personal best My peak flow is between _____ and _____	Action to be taken when in the yellow zone:	Time action taken:	Did it help? No. Now I should …?
Red Zone My rescue medicine is not helping within 15–20 minutes I am wheezing and/or my breathing is hard and fast My lips and/or fingernails are blue I am having difficulty walking and/or talking	Below 50% of my personal best My peak flow is below ______	Action to be taken when in the red zone:	Time action taken:	Did it help? No. Now I should …?

School/Sports Plan

The goal of asthma management is gaining and maintaining control so that the individual can lead a normal, active life. Students with controlled asthma can attend school and participate in sports without fear of their condition interfering. However, teachers, coaches, and school administrators should be made aware of the student's condition and informed of the proper steps to take should an asthma attack occur. Even if the school district has a school nurse program and/or an asthma response program/plan, it is a good idea to have a written plan and information available in the event of an emergency. See Table 7.2 for a sample school/sports plan.

TABLE 7.2 Sample School/Sports Plan

<table>
<tr><td>Name:</td><td>Age:</td><td>School:</td><td>Homeroom teacher:

Grade:</td></tr>
<tr><td>Parent/guardian:</td><td colspan="2">Address:</td><td>Phone:</td></tr>
<tr><td>Parent/guardian:</td><td colspan="2">Address:</td><td>Phone:</td></tr>
<tr><td>Physician:</td><td colspan="2">Address:</td><td>Phone:</td></tr>
<tr><td>Clinic/emergency room preference:</td><td colspan="2">Address:</td><td>Phone:</td></tr>
<tr><td colspan="4">Allergies:</td></tr>
<tr><td colspan="4">Activity restrictions:</td></tr>
<tr><td colspan="4">My asthma triggers are:</td></tr>
<tr><td colspan="4">Emergency steps should be taken when:
My symptoms are:
My peak flow is below:</td></tr>
</table>

TABLE 7.2 Sample School/Sports Plan *(Cont.)*

<table>
<tr><td colspan="2">If I am having difficulty breathing/coughing excessively:
Check my peak flow rate.</td><td>Green zone: My peak flow is above: ____________.
I am okay, but I will need to be checked again.
Yellow zone: My peak flow is between _________ and _____.
Give this medication: ______________.
I should be better in 15–20 minutes. If not, seek assistance.
Red zone: My peak flow is below: ________.
I need immediate emergency help.</td></tr>
<tr><td colspan="3">Contact my parent/guardian if/when:</td></tr>
<tr><td colspan="3">My medications are kept (circle one): with my teacher; with the school nurse; with me; other:</td></tr>
<tr><td>My daily medication plan is:</td><td>Medication</td><td>Dosage/timing</td></tr>
<tr><td>My daily monitoring plan is:</td><td>Peak flow measurement times:</td><td>Symptom checks:</td></tr>
<tr><td>My emergency medication plan is:</td><td>Medication</td><td>Dosage/timing</td></tr>
<tr><td colspan="3">Additional instructions:</td></tr>
<tr><td colspan="3">Parent/guardian signature:

Date:</td></tr>
</table>

Some school systems require a physician's signature for the administration of medications on school property. If that is required, a permission sheet such as the one shown in Table 7.3 can be used to accompany the preceding form.

TABLE 7.3 School Asthma Medication Permission Sheet

<table>
<tr><td>Name:</td><td>Age:</td><td>School:</td><td>Homeroom teacher:

Grade:</td></tr>
<tr><td>Parent/guardian:</td><td colspan="2">Address:</td><td>Phone:</td></tr>
<tr><td>Physician:</td><td colspan="2">Address:</td><td>Phone:</td></tr>
<tr><td colspan="4">To be completed by physician:</td></tr>
<tr><td colspan="4">____________________________ is a patient under my care and has been instructed in the proper way to use his/her asthma medications. It is my professional opinion that ____________________________ should be allowed to carry and use that medication by him/herself on school property and in accordance with school policy.</td></tr>
<tr><td colspan="4">It is my professional opinion that _______________ should not carry his/her asthma medication and may require assistance with these medications.</td></tr>
<tr><td colspan="4">Student requires monitoring/peak flow assistance: yes/no</td></tr>
<tr><td colspan="4">Physician signature:

Date:</td></tr>
<tr><td colspan="4">Parent/guardian signature:

Date:</td></tr>
</table>

Travel Plan

Whether an individual is a student or an adult, organizing his or her health information when traveling is important. Filling out this form and also leaving a copy with a healthcare provider or emergency contact prior to departure can provide useful documentation in the event of an emergency. The form shown in Table 7.4 can be useful when preparing to take a trip.

TABLE 7.4 Asthma Travel Plan

<table>
<tr><td colspan="3">Name:</td></tr>
<tr><td colspan="3">Address:</td></tr>
<tr><td colspan="3">Home phone:</td></tr>
<tr><td colspan="3">Emergency contact:</td></tr>
<tr><td>Physician:</td><td colspan="2">Physician's phone/address:</td></tr>
<tr><td colspan="3">Hospital/clinic preference:</td></tr>
<tr><td colspan="3">Allergies:</td></tr>
<tr><td colspan="3">Diagnosis:</td></tr>
<tr><td colspan="3">I am traveling to/staying with:</td></tr>
<tr><td colspan="3">Insurance company/health provider:</td></tr>
<tr><td colspan="3">Policy/group number:</td></tr>
<tr><td colspan="3">Authorization phone number:</td></tr>
<tr><td>Circle one:</td><td colspan="2">I have advance directives (living will).
Attached. Located:
I have no advance directives.</td></tr>
<tr><td>Circle as needed:</td><td colspan="2">I use oxygen: ___________ lpm
I am an organ donor.
I am an eye donor.</td></tr>
<tr><td colspan="3">My asthma medications are:</td></tr>
<tr><td>Green Zone
No coughing or wheezing
I slept through the night
I can work/play without difficulty</td><td>80%–100% of my personal best
My peak flow is above ______</td><td>Action to be taken when in the green zone:</td></tr>
<tr><td>Yellow Zone
I am getting a cold/infection
I have been exposed to a known trigger/allergen
I am coughing
I am wheezing
I have tightness in my chest
My asthma woke me up last night</td><td>50%–80% of my personal best
My peak flow is between _____ and _____</td><td>Action to be taken when in the yellow zone:</td></tr>
</table>

(continues)

TABLE 7.4 Asthma Travel Plan (*Cont.*)

<table>
<tr><td colspan="2">Red Zone
My rescue medicine is not helping within 15–20 minutes
I am wheezing and/or my breathing is hard and fast
My lips and/or fingernails are blue
I am having difficulty walking and/or talking</td><td colspan="2">Below 50% of my personal best
My peak flow is below
______</td><td>Action to be taken when in the red zone:</td></tr>
<tr><td colspan="5">Other medications I am taking:</td></tr>
<tr><td>Medication:</td><td>Dosage:</td><td>Time:</td><td>Side effects:</td><td>Reason I am taking this medication:</td></tr>
<tr><td></td><td></td><td></td><td></td><td></td></tr>
<tr><td></td><td></td><td></td><td></td><td></td></tr>
<tr><td></td><td></td><td></td><td></td><td></td></tr>
<tr><td></td><td></td><td></td><td></td><td></td></tr>
<tr><td></td><td></td><td></td><td></td><td></td></tr>
<tr><td></td><td></td><td></td><td></td><td></td></tr>
<tr><td colspan="5">Additional information:</td></tr>
</table>

Patient Education

In addition to developing the preceding documents, patient self-management skills and education plays a critical role in gaining and maintaining control of asthma. The development of a partnership between the healthcare providers and the individual has been shown to be an effective strategy for improving asthma outcomes.[1] Whenever possible it is important to include the asthmatic individual in the decision-making process and the development of a written asthma action plan. The components of a successful asthma education plan include:

- The individual's ability to demonstrate an understanding of their triggers and symptoms
- A discussion/implementation of action steps to minimize environmental triggers
- The individual's ability to demonstrate proper technique when taking their medications and completing their self-monitoring (peak flow, symptoms scores, etc.)
- A written asthma action jointly developed by the practitioner and the individual
- An emergency plan that clearly outlines the steps to take when asthma symptoms are not responding to the written asthma action plan steps

There are multiple opportunities and teaching moments that present themselves when managing an asthmatic individual. The patient's education level and medication techniques should be assessed and verified on follow-up visits and periodically throughout the course of their management. Formal outlined education sessions are not necessary; however, it is necessary to insure and document that their skill levels, written asthma action plan, and education are being addressed.

References

1. National Heart, Lung, and Blood Institute. National Asthma Education and Prevention Program Expert Panel Report 3: Guidelines for the Diagnosis and Management of Asthma Full Report 2007. http://www.nhlbi.nih.gov/guidelines/asthma/asthsumm.pdf. Accessed April 2, 2009.
2. The Global Initiative for Asthma (GINA). 2009 Update of the GINA Report, Global Strategy for Asthma Management and Prevention. http://www.ginasthma.com. Accessed April 1, 2010.

8 Stepwise Management for Children 0–4 Years of Age

LEARNING OBJECTIVES

- Discuss stepwise management for the control of asthma therapy in children 0–4 years of age.
- Review the management differences between intermittent and persistent asthma.
- Identify the recommended medication dosages for the treatment of asthma.

KEY WORDS

stepwise management
asthma action plan
components of severity
classification of asthma severity

Introduction

Managing asthma in children 0–4 years of age can be challenging because these children cannot articulate their symptoms and often may be too young to follow treatment instructions. Clinicians must rely on the child's parents/caregivers and immediate family members to help them monitor, assess, and treat the child's asthma. The development of a partnership between the clinician and the child's primary care provider will facilitate guided self-management and the ability to control the child's asthma. This guided self-management is achieved via the written asthma care plan. The chart illustrated in Table 8.1 can assess asthma severity and starting therapy.

TABLE 8.1 Assessing Asthma Control in Children Ages 0–4 Years and Starting Therapy

		Classification/Level of Asthma Severity (0–4 years of age)			
			Persistent		
Components of Severity		*Intermittent*	*Mild*	*Moderate*	*Severe*
Impairment	Symptoms	≤ 2 days per week	> 2 days per week, but not daily	Daily	Throughout the day
	Nighttime awakenings	None	1–2×/month	3–4×/month	> 1×/week
	Short-acting $beta_2$-agonist use for symptom control (not prevention of EIB)	≤ 2 days per week	> 2 days per week, but not daily	Daily	Several times per day
	Interference with normal activity	None	Minor limitation	Some limitation	Extremely limited
Risk impairment	Exacerbations requiring oral systemic corticosteroids	0–1/year	≥ 2 exacerbations in 6 months requiring oral systemic corticosteroids, or ≥ 4 wheezing episodes/1 year lasting > 1 day and risk factors for persistent asthma		
		Consider severity and interval since last exacerbation.			
		Frequency and severity may fluctuate over time.			
		Exacerbations of any severity may occur in patients in any severity category.			

(continues)

TABLE 8.1 Assessing Asthma Control in Children Ages 0–4 Years and Starting Therapy *(Cont.)*

	Classification/Level of Asthma Severity (0–4 years of age)			
		Persistent		
Components of Severity	*Intermittent*	*Mild*	*Moderate*	*Severe*
Recommended step initiating therapy (see the following treatment steps)	Step 1	Step 2	Step 3 and consider short course of oral systemic corticosteroids	
	In 2–6 weeks, depending on severity, evaluate level of asthma control that is achieved. If no clear benefit is observed in 4–6 weeks, consider adjusting therapy or alternative diagnoses.			

EIB = exercise-induced bronchospasm; FEV_1 = forced expiratory volume in 1 second; FVC = forced vital capacity

Notes:

- The stepwise approach is meant to assist, not replace, the clinical decision making required to meet individual patient needs.
- The level of control is based on the most severe impairment or risk category. Assess impairment domain by patient's/caregiver's recall of previous 2–4 weeks and by spirometry/or peak flow measures. Symptom assessment for longer periods should reflect a global assessment such as inquiring whether the patient's asthma is better or worse since the last visit.
- At present, there is inadequate data to correspond frequencies of exacerbations with different levels of asthma control. In general, more frequent and intense exacerbations (e.g., requiring urgent, unscheduled care, hospitalization, or ICU admission) indicate poorer disease control. For treatment purposes, patients who had ≥ 2 exacerbations requiring oral systemic corticosteroids in the past year may be considered the same as patients who have persistent asthma, even in the absence of impairment levels consistent with persistent asthma.
- Before step up in therapy:
  - Review adherence to medications, inhaler technique, environmental control, and comorbid conditions.
  - If alternative treatment option was used in a step, discontinue it and use preferred treatment for that step.

Adapted from: National Heart, Lung, and Blood Institute. National Asthma Education and Prevention Program Expert Panel Report 3: Guidelines for the Diagnosis and Management of Asthma Full Report 2007. http://www.nhlbi.nih.gov/guidelines/asthma/asthsumm.pdf. Accessed April 2, 2009.

Stepwise Management for Children 0–4 Years of Age

Once therapy has been started, a stepwise management plan can guide clinicians in their progressive stepping up or stepping down of treatment as needed. The steps are based on the severity of asthma at the time and it is intended that the lowest dose possible of medication be used when managing a child's asthma. The chart shown in Table 8.2 can assist in determining the level of asthma control and severity.

The six steps presented in the stepwise management plan are designed to assist the clinician in making decisions about the level of care needed. These steps should not be confused with zone recommendations in the patient's asthma action plan. It is possible for patients to have a different asthma action plan based on their current level of severity and step of care. Table 8.3 details the six steps designed to assess asthma therapy.

TABLE 8.2 Assessing Asthma Control in Children Ages 0–4 Years After Therapy Has Been Started

		Classification of Asthma Control (0–4 years of age)		
Components of Control		*Well controlled*	*Not well controlled*	*Very poorly controlled*
Impairment	Symptoms	≤ 2 days per week	> 2 days per week	Throughout the day
	Nighttime awakenings	≤ 1×/month	> 1×/month	> 1×/week
	Interference with normal activity: none, some limitation, or extremely limited	None	Some limitation	Extremely limited
	Short-acting $beta_2$ agonist used for symptom control (not for prevention of EIB)	≤ 2 days per week	> 2 days per week	Several times per day

(continues)

TABLE 8.2 Assessing Asthma Control in Children Ages 0–4 Years After Therapy Has Been Started *(Cont.)*

Risk	Exacerbations requiring oral systemic corticosteroids	0–1×/year	2–3×/year	> 3×/year
	Treatment-related adverse effects	Medication side effects can vary in intensity from none to very troublesome and worrisome. The level of intensity does not correlate to specific levels of control but should be considered in the overall assessment of risk.		

EIB = exercise-induced bronchospasm

Notes:

- The stepwise approach is meant to assist, not replace, the clinical decision making required to meet individual patient needs.
- The level of control is based on the most severe impairment or risk category. Assess impairment domain by caregiver's recall of previous 2–4 weeks. Symptom assessment for longer periods should reflect a global assessment such as inquiring whether the patient's asthma is better or worse since the last visit.
- At present, there are inadequate data to correspond frequencies of exacerbations with different levels of asthma control. In general, more frequent and intense exacerbations (e.g., requiring urgent, unscheduled care, hospitalization, or ICU admission) indicate poorer disease control. For treatment purposes, patients who had ≥ 2 exacerbations requiring oral systemic corticosteroids in the past year may be considered the same as patients who have not-well-controlled asthma, even in the absence of impairment levels consistent with not-well-controlled asthma.
- Before step up in therapy:
  - Review adherence to medications, inhaler technique, and environmental control.
  - If alternative treatment option was used in a step, discontinue it and use preferred treatment for that step.

Adapted from: National Heart, Lung, and Blood Institute. National Asthma Education and Prevention Program Expert Panel Report 3: Guidelines for the Diagnosis and Management of Asthma Full Report 2007. http://www.nhlbi.nih.gov/guidelines/asthma/asthsumm.pdf. Accessed April 2, 2009.

TABLE 8.3 Step Therapy

Intermittent Asthma	*Persistent asthma: daily medication* **Consultation should be considered at Step 2* **An asthma specialist should be consulted if Step 3 care or higher is required*					
Step 1 Preferred reliever: SABA PRN	Step 2 Preferred controllers: low-dose ICS Alternative: cromolyn or montelukast	Step 3 Preferred controllers: medium-dose ICS	Step 4 Preferred controllers: medium-dose ICS + either LABA or montelukast	Step 5 Preferred controllers: high-dose ICS + either LABA or montelukast	Step 6 Preferred controllers: high-dose ICS + either LABA or montelukast Oral systemic corticosteroids	Patient education and environmental control should be assessed at each step

Note: Step 1 is applicable to intermittent asthma. If a child is identified as having persistent asthma, Step 1 reliever medications should be continued and steps 2–6 added based on the severity and level of controller medication needed to gain control.

Step up therapy as needed (first check adherence, inhaler technique, and environmental control). If a medication is started and no clear response occurs within 4–6 weeks, the treatment should be discontinued and an alternative diagnoses and/or other therapy options/adjustments considered.

Step down therapy when possible (asthma is well controlled for at least 3 months). If there is a clear and positive response for at least 3 months, a step down in therapy should be undertaken to the lowest possible doses of medication required to maintain asthma control.

Medication technique and adherence to therapy should be assessed when considering changes in therapy (either up or down) to insure proper technique and that the medication prescribed is being used appropriately.

(continues)

TABLE 8.3 Step Therapy *(Cont.)*

Quick-relief medication for all patients:
SABA as needed for symptoms. Intensity of treatment depends on severity of symptoms.
With viral respiratory infections: SABA q 4–6 hours up to 24 hours (longer with physician consult). Consider short course of oral systemic corticosteroids if exacerbation is severe or patient has history of previous severe exacerbations.
Caution: Frequent use of SABA may indicate the need to step up treatment. See text for recommendations on initiating daily long-term-control therapy.

Alphabetical order is used when more than one treatment option is listed within either preferred or alternative therapy. ICS = inhaled corticosteroid; LABA = inhaled long-acting beta$_2$-agonist; SABA = inhaled short-acting beta$_2$-agonist

Notes: The stepwise approach is meant to assist, not replace, the clinical decision making required to meet individual patient needs.

If alternative treatment is used and response is inadequate, discontinue it and use the preferred treatment before stepping up.

If clear benefit is not observed within 4–6 weeks and patient/family medication technique and adherence are satisfactory, consider adjusting therapy or alternative diagnosis.

Studies on children 0–4 years of age are limited. Step 2 preferred therapy is based on Evidence A. All other recommendations are based on expert opinion and extrapolated from studies in older children.

Adapted from: National Heart, Lung, and Blood Institute. National Asthma Education and Prevention Program Expert Panel Report 3: Guidelines for the Diagnosis and Management of Asthma Full Report 2007. http://www.nhlbi.nih.gov/guidelines/asthma/asthsumm.pdf. Accessed April 2, 2009.

Step 1 Care for Children 0–4 Years of Age

Intermittent Asthma

Intermittent asthma is defined as symptoms occurring less than once a week, brief exacerbations, nocturnal symptoms not more than twice a month, a FEV_1 or PEF of 80% predicted and a PEF or FEV_1 variability < 20%.[1] Intermittent asthma should be assessed regularly to evaluate whether the individual's asthma is indeed intermittent. The occurrence of two or more severe exacerbations within 6 months without symptoms in between is an example of minimal or intermittent impairment, but demonstrates a persistent, high risk of exacerbation. Individuals presenting with this pattern of asthma should be classified as having persistent asthma and may benefit from daily long-term control therapy.

Step one therapy for children 0–4 years of age with intermittent asthma includes the use of SABAs as needed to treat immediate symptoms. The current U.S. guidelines state that reliever medication (SABAs) can be continued indefinitely on an as-needed basis. Increasing usage of these medications, however, may indicate more severe or inadequately controlled asthma. When this occurs a step up in therapy may be needed. A written asthma action plan should be developed for individuals who have intermittent asthma and a history of severe exacerbations. This plan should include measurable signs and symptoms of worsening asthma (either peak flow measurement or specific symptoms), recommendations for using reliever medications, when to begin oral systemic corticosteroids, and detailed information as to when the patient should seek medical assistance. If the child is not adequately controlled with the use of as-needed reliever medications he or she should be reevaluated for persistent asthma.

Persistent Asthma

If a child is identified as having persistent asthma he or she should be considered for Step 2 or higher management. The goal of management is to gain and maintain control with the minimum amount of controller medication necessary. Daily long-term control medication is recommended for these children if they have had four or more wheezing episodes in 1 year and risk factors for persistent asthma. Daily therapy may be needed for children who have had a second exacerbation requiring oral systemic corticosteroids in 6 months or children who consistently require symptomatic treatment > 2 days a week for > 4 weeks. In addition to the controller medication recommendations included in steps 2–6, reliever medication (SABAs) should be available and used as needed to relieve symptoms. See Table 8.4 for the usual dosages for reliever medication in children.

TABLE 8.4 Usual Dosages for Reliever Medication in Children*

Inhaled Short-Acting Beta$_2$ Agonists (SABAs)			
Medication	*Formulation*	*0–4 years*	*Comments*
	MDI		
Albuterol CFC	90 mcg/puff, 200 puffs/ canister	1–2 puffs 5 minutes before exercise	Differences in potencies exist, but all products are essentially comparable on a per puff basis. An increasing use or lack of expected effect indicates diminished control of asthma. Not recommended for long-term daily treatment. Regular use exceeding 2 days/week for symptom control (not prevention of EIB) indicates the need for additional long-term control therapy. May double usual dose for mild exacerbations.
Albuterol HFA	90 mcg/puff, 200 puffs/ canister	2 puffs every 4–6 hours as needed	
Levalbuterol HFA	45 mcg/puff, 200 puffs/ canister	Safety and efficacy not established in children < 4 years of age	Should prime the inhaler by releasing four actuations prior to use. Periodically clean HFA actuator, as drug may plug orifice.

Pirbuterol CFC Autohaler	200 mcg/puff, 400 puffs/ canister	Safety and efficacy not established	Children < 4 years of age may not generate sufficient inspiratory flow to activate an auto-inhaler. Nonselective agents (i.e., epinephrine, isoproterenol, metaproterenol) are not recommended due to their potential for excessive cardiac stimulation, especially in high doses.
Albuterol	**Nebulizer solution** 0.63 mg/3 mL 1.25 mg/3 mL 2.5 mg/3 mL 5 mg/mL (0.5%)	0.63–2.5 mg in 3 cc of saline q 4–6 hours, as needed	May mix with cromolyn solution, budesonide inhalant suspension, or ipratropium solution for nebulization. May double dose for severe exacerbations.
Levalbuterol(R-albuterol)	0.31 mg/3 mL 0.63 mg/3 mL 1.25 mg/0.5 mL 1.25 mg/3 mL	0.31–1.25 mg in 3 cc q 4–6 hours, as needed	Does not have FDA-approved labeling for children < 6 years of age. The product is a sterile-filled, preservative-free, unit dose vial. Compatible with budesonide inhalant suspension.

(continues)

TABLE 8.4 Usual Dosages for Reliever Medication in Children*

	Inhaled Short-Acting Beta$_2$ Agonists (SABAs)		
Medication	*Formulation*	*0–4 years*	*Comments*
Anticholinergics			
Ipratropium HFA	**MDI** 17 mcg/puff, 200 puffs/canister **Nebulizer Solution** 0.25 mg/mL (0.025%)	Safety and efficacy not established Safety and efficacy not established	Evidence is lacking for anticholinergics producing added benefit to beta$_2$-agonists in long-term asthma therapy.
Systemic Corticosteroids			
Methylprednisolone	2, 4, 6, 8, 16, 32 mg tablets	Short course "burst": 1–2 mg/kg/day, maximum 60 mg/day, for 3–10 days	Short courses or "bursts" are effective for establishing control when initiating therapy or during a period of gradual deterioration. The burst should be continued until patient achieves 80% PEF personal best or symptoms resolve. This usually requires 3–10 days but may require a longer treatment period. There is no evidence that tapering the dose following improvement prevents relapse.
Prednisolone	5 mg tablets, 5 mg/5 cc, 15 mg/5 cc		
Prednisone	1, 2.5, 5, 10, 20, 50 mg tablets; 5 mg/cc, 5 mg/5 cc		

Methylprednisolone acetate	**Repository injection** 40 mg/mL 80 mg/mL	7.5 mg/kg IM once	May be used in place of a short burst of oral steroids in patients who are vomiting or if adherence is a problem.

CFC = chlorofluorocarbon; ED = emergency department; EIB = exercise-induced bronchospasm; HFA = hydrofluoroalkane; IM = intramuscular; MDI = metered-dose inhaler; PEF = peak expiratory flow

*Dosages are provided for those products that have been approved by the FDA or that have sufficient clinical trial safety and efficacy data in the appropriate age ranges to support their use.

Adapted from: National Heart, Lung, and Blood Institute. National Asthma Education and Prevention Program Expert Panel Report 3: Guidelines for the Diagnosis and Management of Asthma Full Report 2007. http://www.nhlbi.nih.gov/guidelines/asthma/asthsumm.pdf. Accessed April 2, 2009.

Step 2 Care for Children 0–4 Years of Age

The preferred treatment for children at Step 2 is daily low-dose inhaled corticosteroids (ICS). Alternative therapies that may be considered are cromolyn and montelukast (listed in alphabetical order). If one of these alternative treatments is selected and adequate asthma control is not achieved and maintained in 4–6 weeks, then discontinue that treatment and use the preferred medication before stepping up therapy. Theophylline is not recommended in children less than 5 years of age due to the challenges of serum monitoring and also documented irregularities in theophylline metabolism during febrile illness.

There has been controversy over the use of corticosteroids to treat asthma in children. The current U.S. guidelines state that "the potential for the adverse effect of low- to medium-dose ICS on linear growth is usually limited to a small reduction in growth velocity, approximately 1 cm in the first year of treatment that is generally not progressive over time."[2] They recommend that children receiving ICS should be monitored, by using a stadiometer, for changes in growth. The guidelines also note that "High doses of ICS administered for prolonged periods of time (for example, more than 1 year), particularly in combination with frequent courses of systemic corticosteroid therapy, may be associated with adverse growth effects and risk of posterior subcapsular cataracts or reduced bone density."[2] They recommend that children taking these medications should also have age-appropriate dietary intake of calcium and vitamin D in addition to slit-lamp eye examinations and bone densitometry evaluations. See Table 8.5 for usual dosages of long-term control medication in children.

Step 3 Care for Children 0–4 Years of Age

The current U.S. guidelines recommend increasing the dose of ICS to insure an adequate amount of medication is delivered before adding adjunctive therapy (see Table 8.6). This advancement to medium-dose ICS is intended to offset the potential variability of delivering aerosols to children in this age group, as often they are too young to understand and follow the recommended delivery strategies.

Step 4 Care for Children 0–4 Years of Age

Step 4 should be considered when increasing the dose of the ICS has not been successful in controlling the asthma. In this step the medium dose ICS is continued and adjunctive therapies may be added. These therapies include LABAs and montelukast. As a reminder theophylline is not recommended as an add-on therapy for this age group.

TABLE 8.5 Usual Dosages for Long-Term Control Medication for Children*

Systemic Corticosteroids			
Medication	*Formulation*	*0–4 years*	*Comments*
Methylprednisolone	2, 4, 8, 16, 32 mg tablets	0.25–2 mg/kg daily in single dose in a.m. or qod as needed for control	For long-term treatment of severe persistent asthma, administer single dose in a.m. either daily or on alternate days (alternate-day therapy may produce less adrenal suppression) Short courses or "bursts" are effective for establishing control when initiating therapy or during a period of gradual deterioration.
Prednisolone	5 mg tablets, 5 mg/5 cc, 15 mg/5 cc	Short-course "burst": 1–2 mg/kg/day, maximum 60 mg/day for 3–10 days	There is no evidence that tapering the dose following improvement in symptom control and pulmonary function prevents relapse.
Prednisone	1, 2.5, 5, 10, 20, 50 mg tablets; 5 mg/cc, 5 mg/5 cc	Short-course "burst": 1–2 mg/kg/day, maximum 60 mg/day for 3–10 days	Patients receiving the lower dose (1 mg/kg/day) experience fewer behavioral side effects (Kayani & Shannon, 2002), and it appears to be equally efficacious (Rachelefsky, 2003). For patients unable to tolerate the liquid preparations, dexamethasone syrup at 0.4 mg/kg/day may be an alternative. Studies are limited, however, and the longer duration of activity increases the risk of adrenal suppression (Hendeles, 2003).

(continues)

TABLE 8.5 Usual Dosages for Long-Term Control Medication for Children *(Cont.)*

		Systemic Corticosteroids	
Medication	*Formulation*	*0–4 years*	*Comments*
Long-Acting $Beta_2$ Agonists (LABAs)			
Salmeterol	DPI 50 mcg/ blister	Safety and efficacy not established in children < 4 years of age	Should not be used for symptom relief or exacerbations. Use only with ICS. Salmeterol DPI 50 mcg/blister: safety and efficacy not established in children < 4 years; 1 blister q 12 hours. Decreased duration of protection against EIB may occur with regular use.
Formoterol	DPI 12 mcg/ single-use capsule	Safety and efficacy not established in children < 5 years	Most children < 4 years of age cannot provide sufficient inspiratory flow for adequate lung delivery. Do not blow into inhaler after dose is activated. Formoterol DPI 12 mcg/single-use capsule: safety and efficacy not established in children < 5 years; 1 capsule q 12 hours. Most children < 4 years of age cannot provide sufficient inspiratory flow for adequate lung delivery. Each capsule is for single use only; additional doses should not be administered for at least 12 hours. Capsules should be used only with the inhaler and should not be taken orally.

*Dosages are provided for those products that have been approved by the FDA or have sufficient clinical trial safety and efficacy data in the appropriate age ranges to support their use.

Combined Medications			
Fluticasone/ salmeterol	DPI 100 mcg/50 mcg	Safety and efficacy not established in children < 4 years	There have been no clinical trials in children < 4 years of age. Most children < 4 years of age cannot provide sufficient inspiratory flow for adequate lung delivery. Do not blow into inhaler after dose is activated.
Budesonide/ Formoterol	**HFA MDI** 80 mcg/4.5 mcg	Safety and efficacy not established	There have been no clinical trials in children < 4 years of age. Currently approved for use in youths ≥ 12 years of age. Dose for children 5–12 years of age is based on clinical trials using DPI with slightly different delivery characteristics.
Cromolyn/Nedocromil			
Cromolyn	**MDI** 0.8 mg/puff **Nebulizer** 20 mg/ampule	Safety and efficacy not established 1 ampule qid Safety and efficacy not established < 2 years	Four to six week trial may be needed to determine maximum benefit. Dose by MDI may be inadequate to affect hyperresponsiveness. One dose before exercise or allergen exposure provides effective prophylaxis for 1–2 hours. Not as effective as inhaled $beta_2$-agonists for EIB. Once control is achieved, the frequency of dosing may be reduced.
Nedocromil	**MDI** 1.75 mg/puff	Safety and efficacy not established < 6 years	

(continues)

TABLE 8.5 Usual Dosages for Long-Term Control Medication for Children *(Cont.)*

		Systemic Corticosteroids	
Medication	*Formulation*	*0–4 years*	*Comments*
Leukotriene Receptor Antagonists (LTRAs)			
Montelukast	4 mg or 5 mg chewable tablet 4 mg granule packets	4 mg qhs (1–5 years of age)	Montelukast exhibits a flat dose response curve. No more efficacious than placebo in infants 6–24 months. For zafirlukast, administration with meals decreases bioavailability; take at least 1 hour before or 2 hours after meals. Monitor for signs and symptoms of hepatic dysfunction.
Zafirlukast	10 mg tablet	Safety and efficacy not established	
Methylxanthines			
Theophylline	Liquids, sustained-release tablets, and capsules	Starting dose 10 mg/kg/day; Usual maximum: < 1 year of age: 0.2 (age in weeks) + 5 = mg/kg/day; ≥ 1 year of age = 16 mg/kg/day	Adjust dosage to achieve serum concentration of 5–15 mcg/mL at steady-state (at least 48 hours on same dosage). Due to wide interpatient variability in theophylline metabolic clearance, routine serum theophylline level monitoring is essential. See additional information in this chapter for factors that can affect theophylline levels.

DPI = dry-powder inhaler; EIB = exercise-induced bronchospasm; HFA = hydrofluoroalkane (inhaler propellant); MDI = metered-dose inhaler

Adapted from: National Heart, Lung, and Blood Institute. National Asthma Education and Prevention Program Expert Panel Report 3: Guidelines for the Diagnosis and Management of Asthma Full Report 2007. http://www.nhlbi.nih.gov/guidelines/asthma/asthsumm.pdf. Accessed April 2, 2009.

TABLE 8.6 Estimated Comparative Daily Dosages for Inhaled Corticosteroids in Children 0–4 Years of Age

Drug	*Low Daily Dose*	*Medium Daily Dose*	*High Daily Dose*
Beclomethasone HFA 40 or 80 mcg/puff	NA	NA	NA
Budesonide DPI 90, 180, or 200 mcg/inhalation	NA	NA	NA
Budesonide inhaled Inhalation suspension for nebulization (child dose)	0.25–0.5 mg	> 0.5–1.0 mg	> 1.0 mg
Flunisolide 250 mcg/puff	NA	NA	NA
Flunisolide HFA 80 mcg/puff	NA	NA	NA
Fluticasone HFA/MDI 44, 110, or 220 mcg/puff	176 mcg	> 176–352 mcg	> 352 mcg
DPI: 50, 100, or 250 mcg/inhalation	NA	NA	NA
Mometasone DPI 200 mcg/inhalation	NA	NA	NA
Triamcinolone acetonide 75 mcg/puff	NA	NA	NA

HFA = hydrofluoroalkane; NA = not approved and/or no data available for this age group

Notes: The most important determinant of appropriate dosing is the clinician's judgment of the patient's response to therapy. The clinician must monitor the patient's response on several clinical parameters and adjust the dose accordingly. The stepwise approach to therapy emphasizes that once control of asthma is achieved, the dose of medication should be carefully titrated to the minimum dose required to maintain control, thus reducing the potential for adverse effect.

Some doses may be outside package labeling, especially in the high-dose range. Budesonide nebulizer suspension is the only ICS with FDA approved labeling for children < 4 years of age.

Metered-dose inhaler (MDI) dosages are expressed as the actuator dose (the amount of the drug leaving the actuator and delivered to the patient), which is the labeling required in the United States. This is different from the dosage expressed as the valve dose (the amount of

(continues)

TABLE 8.6 Estimated Comparative Daily Dosages for Inhaled Corticosteroids in Children 0–4 Years of Age *(Cont.)*

drug leaving the valve, not all of which is available to the patient), which is used in many European countries and in some scientific literature. Dry-powder inhaler (DPI) doses are expressed as the amount of drug in the inhaler following activation.

For children < 4 years of age: the safety and efficacy of ICS in children < 1 year have not been established. Children < 4 years of age generally require delivery of ICS (budesonide and fluticasone HFA) through a face mask that should fit snugly over nose and mouth and avoid nebulizing in the eyes. Wash face after each treatment to prevent local corticosteroid side effects. For budesonide, the dose may be administered 1–3 times daily. Budesonide suspension is compatible with albuterol, ipratropium, and levalbuterol nebulizer solutions in the same nebulizer. Use only jet nebulizers, as ultrasonic nebulizers are ineffective for suspensions.

For fluticasone HFA, the dose should be divided 2 times daily; the low dose for children < 4 years is higher than for children 5–11 years of age due to lower dose delivered with face mask and data on efficacy in young children.

Adapted from: National Heart, Lung, and Blood Institute. National Asthma Education and Prevention Program Expert Panel Report 3: Guidelines for the Diagnosis and Management of Asthma Full Report 2007. Available http://www.nhlbi.nih.gov/guidelines/asthma/asthsumm.pdf. Accessed April 2, 2009.

Step 5 Care for Children 0–4 Years of Age

Increasing the dose of ICS to a high level and using either a LABA or montelukast is the preferred treatment at Step 5. See Table 8.7 for long-term control medications for children.

TABLE 8.7 Long-Term Control Medications Approved by the Food and Drug Administration for Children

Inhaled corticosteroids (ICS)	Budesonide nebulizer solution (approved for children 1–8 years of age) Fluticasone DPI (approved for children 4 years of age and older)
Long-acting inhaled beta$_2$-agonist (LABA)	Salmeterol DPI and combination product (salmeterol + fluticasone) DPI (approved for children 4 years of age and older)
Leukotriene receptor antagonists (LTRA)	Montelukast, 4 mg chewable tablet (approved for children 2–6 years of age) and 4 mg granules (approved for 1 year of age and older)
Mast cell inhibitors	Cromolyn nebulizer (approved for children ≥ 2 years of age)

Step 6 Care for Children 0–4 Years of Age

Step 6 includes the use of high-dose ICS and either LABA or montelukast, in addition to oral systemic corticosteroids. It is a good idea to complete a 2-week course of oral systemic corticosteroids to confirm clinical reversibility and an effective response to therapy when starting oral corticosteroids. If the child is 4 years of age or older, high-dose ICS in combination with both an LTRA and a LABA may also be an option. When administering long-term oral systemic corticosteroids, the lowest dose possible to achieve control should be used. Single daily dosing and/or alternative day dosing may be an option for this age group. For management purposes high doses of ICS are the preferred therapy because they have fewer side effects than oral systemic corticosteroids. See Table 8.8 for recommended considerations when using corticosteroids in children.

Stepping Up and Stepping Down

The current U.S. guidelines acknowledge that treatment recommendations are based on limited data in this age group, and that determining treatment schedules is often done via a therapeutic trial in each individual case. For this reason close monitoring of the child's response to therapy is encouraged. If a medication is started and no clear response occurs within 4–6 weeks the treatment should be discontinued and an alternative diagnosis therapy option reviewed. If there is a clear and positive response for at least 3 months, a step down in therapy should be undertaken to the lowest possible doses of medication required to maintain asthma control. Medication technique and adherence to therapy should also be assessed when considering changes in therapy to insure proper technique and that the medication prescribed is being used appropriately.

Follow-Up Visits

While the frequency of visits for review of asthma control is a matter of clinical judgment, in general, individuals who have intermittent or mild persistent asthma that has been under control for at least 3 months should be

TABLE 8.8 Long-Term Oral Systemic Corticosteroid Management

Use the lowest possible dose to achieve control.
Monitor patients closely for adverse effects.
Reduce oral systemic corticosteroids as soon as control is achieved.
Recommend consultation with an asthma specialist.

seen about every 6 months. Individuals who have uncontrolled and/or severe persistent asthma and those who need additional supervision should be seen more often.

Viral Infections

Viral infections are very common in children under 5 years of age and can trigger asthma symptoms. Reliever medications (SABAs) can be used to treat symptoms in children with asthma. If the child's asthma symptoms are mild, treatment with the SABA every 4–6 hours for 24 hours may be sufficient to control symptoms and improve lung function. If this does not relieve the symptoms then further evaluation/consultation should be considered. If the child is having a recurrence of symptoms more than every 6 weeks, they should be considered for a step up to long-term care. If the child's symptoms are moderate-to-severe, a short course of oral systemic corticosteroids should be considered (1 mg/kg/day prednisone or equivalent for 3–10 days). In children who have a history of severe exacerbations in response to viral respiratory infections, oral systemic corticosteroids should be considered at the first sign of the infection.

TABLE 8.9 Special Considerations for Managing Asthma Exacerbations in Infants

Assessment depends on physical examination rather than objective measurements. Use of accessory muscles, inspiratory and expiratory wheezing, paradoxical breathing, cyanosis, and a respiratory rate > 60 are key signs of serious distress.
Objective measurements, such as oxygen saturation (SaO_2) of < 90%, also indicate serious distress.
Response to SABA therapy can be variable and may not be a reliable predictor of satisfactory outcome. However, because infants are at greater risk for respiratory failure, a lack of response noted by either physical examination or objective measurements should be an indication for hospitalization.
Use of oral systemic corticosteroids early in the episode is essential but should not substitute for careful assessment by a physician.
Most acute wheezing episodes result from viral infections and may be accompanied by fever. Antibiotics generally are not required.

SABA = short-acting beta$_2$-agonist

Adapted from: National Heart, Lung, and Blood Institute. National Asthma Education and Prevention Program Expert Panel Report 3: Guidelines for the Diagnosis and Management of Asthma Full Report 2007. http://www.nhlbi.nih.gov/guidelines/asthma/asthsumm.pdf. Accessed April 2, 2009.

Once the child's symptoms are relieved the SABA use can be continued on an as-needed basis and he or she can be returned to their previous management plan.

References

1. The Global Initiative for Asthma (GINA). 2009 Update of the GINA Report, Global Strategy for Asthma Management and Prevention. http://www.ginasthma.com. Accessed April 1, 2009.
2. National Heart, Lung, and Blood Institute. National Asthma Education and Prevention Program Expert Panel Report 3: Guidelines for the Diagnosis and Management of Asthma Full Report 2007. http://www.nhlbi.nih.gov/guidelines/asthma/asthsumm.pdf. Accessed April 2, 2009.

9

Managing Asthma in Children 5–11 Years of Age

LEARNING OBJECTIVES

- Discuss stepwise management for the control of asthma therapy in children 5–11 years of age.
- Review the management differences between intermittent and persistent asthma.
- Identify the recommended medication dosages for the treatment of asthma in children 5–11 years of age.

KEY WORDS

stepwise management
asthma action plan
components of severity
classification of asthma severity

Introduction

Managing asthma in children 5–11 years of age requires the development of a partnership between the medical provider, the parents, school authorities, and the child. A written asthma action plan and school plan should be developed and kept up-to-date to insure the minimal risk of exacerbation.

Selecting Initial Therapy

The selection of initial therapy for children 5–11 years of age should be based on an assessment of the child's classification of severity and degree of impairment as well as the potential risk they face for further exacerbations. Table 9.1 can assist in weighing these factors.[1]

TABLE 9.1 Assessing Asthma Control and Starting Therapy in Children Ages 5–11 Years

		Classification of Asthma Severity (5–11 years of age)			
			Persistent		
Components of Severity		*Intermittent*	*Mild*	*Moderate*	*Severe*
Impairment	Symptoms	≤ 2 days per week	> 2 days per week but not daily	Daily	Throughout the day
	Nighttime awakenings	≤ 2×/month	3–4×/month	> 1×/week but not nightly	Often 7×/week
	Short-acting $beta_2$-agonist use for symptom control (not prevention of EIB)	≤ 2 days per week	> 2 days per week but not daily	Daily	Several times per day
	Interference with normal activity	None	Minor limitation	Some limitation	Extremely limited
Risk impairment	Exacerbations requiring oral systemic corticosteroids	0–1×/year (see note)	≥ 2 per year (see note)		
		Consider severity and interval since last exacerbation.			
		Frequency and severity may fluctuate over time for patients in any severity category.			
		Relative annual risk of exacerbations may be related to FEV_1.			

(continues)

TABLE 9.1 Assessing Asthma Control and Starting Therapy in Children Ages 5–11 Years *(Cont.)*

	Classification of Asthma Severity (5–11 years of age)			
		Persistent		
Components of Severity	*Intermittent*	*Mild*	*Moderate*	*Severe*
Recommended step initiating therapy (see the following treatment steps)	Step 1	Step 2	Step 3: medium dose ICS option and consider short course of oral systemic corticosteroids	Step 3: medium-dose ICS option, or step 4 and consider short course of oral systemic corticosteroids
	In 2–6 weeks, evaluate level of asthma control that is achieved and adjust therapy accordingly.			

EIB = exercise-induced bronchospasm; FEV_1 = forced expiratory volume in 1 second; FVC = forced vital capacity; ICS = inhaled corticosteroids

Notes:

- The stepwise approach is meant to assist, not replace, the clinical decision making required to meet individual patient needs.
- Level of severity is determined by both impairment and risk. Assess impairment domain by patient's/caregiver's recall of the previous 2–4 weeks and spirometry. Assign severity to the most severe category in which any feature occurs.
- At present, there is inadequate data to correspond frequencies of exacerbations with different levels of asthma severity. In general, more frequent and intense exacerbations (e.g., requiring urgent, unscheduled care, hospitalization, or ICU admission) indicate greater underlying disease severity. For treatment purposes, patients who had ≥ 2 exacerbations requiring oral systemic corticosteroids in the past year may be considered the same as patients who have persistent asthma, even in the absence of impairment levels consistent with patients who have persistent asthma.

Adapted from: National Heart, Lung, and Blood Institute. National Asthma Education and Prevention Program Expert Panel Report 3: Guidelines for the Diagnosis and Management of Asthma Full Report 2007. http://www.nhlbi.nih.gov/guidelines/asthma/asthsumm.pdf. Accessed April 2, 2009.

TABLE 9.2 Usual Dosages for Reliever Medication in Children 5–11 Years of Age*

Inhaled short-acting beta$_2$-agonists

Medication	*Formulation*	*5–11 years*	*Comments*
	MDI		Differences in potencies exist, but all products are essentially comparable on a per puff basis.
Albuterol CFC	90 mcg/puff, 200 puffs/canister	1–2 puffs 5 minutes before exercise	An increasing use or lack of expected effect indicates diminished control of asthma.
Albuterol HFA	90 mcg/puff, 200 puffs/canister	2 puffs every 4–6 hours as needed	Not recommended for long-term daily treatment. Regular use exceeding 2 days/week for symptom control (not prevention of EIB) indicates the need for additional long-term control therapy. May double usual dose for mild exacerbations.
Levalbuterol HFA	45 mcg/puff, 200 puffs/canister	2 puffs every 4–6 hours as needed	Should prime the inhaler by releasing 4 actuations prior to use. Periodically clean HFA actuator, as drug may plug orifice.
Pirbuterol CFC Autohaler	200 mcg/puff, 400 puffs/canister	Safety and efficacy not established	Children < 4 years of age may not generate sufficient inspiratory flow to activate an auto-inhaler. Nonselective agents (i.e., epinephrine, isoproterenol, taproterenol) are not recommended due to their potential for excessive cardiac stimulation, especially in high doses.

(continues)

TABLE 9.2 Usual Dosages for Reliever Medication in Children 5–11 Years of Age *(Cont.)*

Inhaled short-acting beta$_2$-agonists			
Medication	*Formulation*	*5–11 years*	*Comments*
Albuterol	**Nebulizer solution**		May mix with cromolyn solution, budesonide inhalant suspension, or ipratropium solution for nebulization.
	0.63 mg/3 mL 1.25 mg/3 mL 2.5 mg/3 mL 5 mg/mL (0.5%)	1.25–5 mg in 3 cc of saline q 4–8 hours, as needed	May double dose for severe exacerbations.
Levalbuterol (R-albuterol)	0.31 mg/3 mL 0.63 mg/3 mL 1.25 mg/0.5 mL 1.25 mg/3 mL	0.31–0.63 mg, q 8 hours, as needed	Does not have FDA-approved labeling for children < 6 years of age. The product is a sterile-filled, preservative-free unit dose vial. Compatible with budesonide inhalant suspension.
Anticholinergics			
Ipratropium HFA	**MDI**		Evidence is lacking for anticholinergics producing added benefit to beta$_2$-agonists in long-term control asthma therapy.
	17 mcg/puff, 200 puffs/canister	Safety and efficacy not established	
	Nebulizer Solution	Safety and efficacy not established	
	0.25 mg/mL (0.025%)		

Systemic corticosteroids			
Methylprednisolone	2, 4, 6, 8, 16, 32 mg tablets	Short course "burst": 1–2 mg/kg/day, maximum 60 mg/day, for 3–10 days	Short courses or "bursts" are effective for establishing control when initiating therapy or during a period of gradual deterioration. The burst should be continued until patient achieves 80% PEF personal best or symptoms resolve. This usually requires 3–10 days but may require a longer treatment period. There is no evidence that tapering the dose following improvement prevents relapse.
Prednisolone	5 mg tablets, 5 mg/5 cc, 15 mg/5 cc		
Prednisone	1, 2.5, 5, 10, 20, 50 mg tablets; 5 mg/cc, 5 mg/5 cc		
	Repository injection		
Methylprednisolone acetate	40 mg/mL 80 mg/mL	240 mg IM once	May be used in place of a short burst of oral steroids in patients who are vomiting or if adherence is a problem.

CFC = chlorofluorocarbon; ED = emergency department; EIB = exercise-induced bronchospasm; HFA = hydrofluoroalkane; IM = intramuscular; MDI = metered-dose inhaler; PEF = peak expiratory flow

*Dosages are provided for those products that have been approved by the FDA or have sufficient clinical trial safety and efficacy data in the appropriate age ranges to support their use.

Adapted from: National Heart, Lung, and Blood Institute. National Asthma Education and Prevention Program Expert Panel Report 3: Guidelines for the Diagnosis and Management of Asthma Full Report 2007. http://www.nhlbi.nih.gov/guidelines/asthma/asthsumm.pdf. Accessed April 2, 2009.

Reliever medication should be selected at a level that achieves asthma control. Just as in younger children, the lowest dose needed to achieve control should be used. The recommended dosages for reliever medication in children ages 5–11 years are listed in Table 9.2.

Daily inhaled corticosteroids are the preferred therapy for persistent asthma. Alternative therapies for this age group include cromolyn, LTRAs, and theophylline. When initiating daily long-term control therapy, the possible long-term adverse side effects of the medication should be compared to the potential risk of uncontrolled asthma. Data suggests that the use of ICS for the control of asthma improves health in children who have mild or moderate persistent asthma. There is a potential small risk of delayed growth from the use of ICS; however, the current U.S. guidelines recommend that this risk is well balanced by the medications effectiveness.[1] Long-term data shows that most children treated with the recommended doses of ICS achieve their predicted adult heights.[2] The recommended dosages of controller medications for children ages 5–11 are listed in Table 9.3.

Stepwise Management

A stepwise management plan can guide clinicians in their progressive stepping up or stepping down of therapy as needed. The steps are based on the severity of asthma at the time, and it is intended that the lowest dose possible of medication be used when managing a child's asthma. Table 9.4 can assist in determining the level of asthma control and severity.

Step 1 Care for Children 5–11 Years of Age

Intermittent Asthma

Reliever medications, specifically SABAs, are the preferred therapy for intermittent asthma. If the child requires increasing dosages or their symptoms aren't controlled by the reliever medication, they should be assessed for persistent asthma. A short course of oral systemic corticosteroids should be considered for children with intermittent asthma who experience moderate or severe exacerbations associated with viral infections. Starting corticosteroids may be considered for children with a history of severe exacerbations due to infections. The child's written asthma action plan should include specific symptoms and PEF levels that alert them to changes in their condition and steps to take when these changes occur. The U.S. guidelines classify a child who experiences more than two exacerbations per year that require oral systemic corticosteroids, even though there may be no symptoms in between the exacerbations, as having minimal or intermittent impairment, but are at a persistent risk of exacerbation. This child should be considered to have persistent asthma and managed as such.

TABLE 9.3 Usual Dosages for Long-Term Control Medication in Children 5–11 Years of Age*

Systemic Corticosteroids			
Medication	*Formulation*	*5–11 years*	*Comments*
Methylprednisolone	2, 4, 8, 16, 32 mg tablets	0.25–2 mg/kg daily in single dose in a.m. or qod as needed for control	For long-term treatment of severe persistent asthma, administer single dose in a.m. either daily or on alternate days (alternate-day therapy may produce less adrenal suppression).
Prednisolone	5 mg tablets, 5 mg/5 cc, 15 mg/5 cc	Short-course "burst": 1–2 mg/kg/day, maximum 60 mg/day for 3–10 days	Short courses or "bursts" are effective for establishing control when initiating therapy or during a period of gradual deterioration. There is no evidence that tapering the dose following improvement in symptom control and pulmonary function prevents relapse.
Prednisone	1, 2.5, 5, 10, 20, 50 mg tablets; 5 mg/cc, 5 mg/5 cc	Short-course "burst": 1–2 mg/kg/day, maximum 60 mg/day for 3–10 days	Patients receiving the lower dose (1 mg/kg/day) experience fewer behavioral side effects and it appears to be equally efficacious. For patients unable to tolerate the liquid preparations, dexamethasone syrup at 0.4 mg/kg/day may be an alternative. Studies are limited, however, and the longer duration of activity increases the risk of adrenal suppression.

(continues)

TABLE 9.3 Usual Dosages for Long-Term Control Medication in Children 5–11 Years of Age *(Cont.)*

		Systemic Corticosteroids	
Medication	*Formulation*	*5–11 years*	*Comments*
Long-acting beta$_2$-agonists (LABAs)			
Salmeterol	**DPI** 50 mcg/blister	1 blister q 12 hours	Should not be used for symptom relief or exacerbations. Use only with ICS.
Formoterol	**DPI** 12 mcg/single-use capsule	1 capsule q 12 hours	Salmeterol DPI 50 mcg/blister: safety and efficacy not established in children < 4 years Decreased duration of protection against EIB may occur with regular use. Most children < 4 years of age cannot provide sufficient inspiratory flow for adequate lung delivery. Do not blow into inhaler after dose is activated. Formoterol DPI 12 mcg/single-use capsule: safety and efficacy not established in children < 5 years Most children < 4 years of age cannot provide sufficient inspiratory flow for adequate lung delivery. Each capsule is for single use only; additional doses should not be administered for at least 12 hours. Capsules should be used only with the inhaler and should not be taken orally.

*Dosages are provided for those products that have been approved by the FDA or have sufficient clinical trial safety and efficacy data in the appropriate age ranges to support their use.

Medication	*Formulation*	*5–11 years*	*Comments*
Combined medication			
Fluticasone/ Salmeterol	**DPI** 100 mcg/50 mcg	1 inhalation bid	There have been no clinical trials in children < 4 years of age. Most children < 4 years of age cannot provide sufficient inspiratory flow for adequate lung delivery. Do not blow into inhaler after dose is activated.
Budesonide/ Formoterol	**HFA MDI** 80 mcg/4.5 mcg	2 puffs bid	There have been no clinical trials in children < 4 years of age. Currently approved for use in youths ≥ 1. Dose for children 5–11 years of age based on clinical trials using DPI with slightly different delivery characteristics.
Cromolyn/nedocromil			
Cromolyn	**MDI** 0.8 mg/puff **Nebulizer** 20 mg/ampule	2 puffs qid 1 ampule qid	4–6 week trial may be needed to determine maximum benefit. Dose by MDI may be inadequate to affect hyperresponsiveness. One dose before exercise or allergen exposure provides effective prophylaxis for 1–2 hours. Not as effective as inhaled $beta_2$-agonists for EIB. Once control is achieved, the frequency of dosing may be reduced.
Nedocromil	**MDI** 1.75 mg/puff	2 puffs qid	

(continues)

TABLE 9.3 Usual Dosages for Long-Term Control Medication in Children 5–11 Years of Age *(Cont.)*

Systemic Corticosteroids			
Medication	*Formulation*	*5–11 years*	*Comments*
Leukotriene receptor antagonists (LTRAs)			
Montelukast	4 mg or 5 mg chewable tablet 4 mg granule packets	5 mg qhs (6–14 years of age)	Montelukast exhibits a flat dose response curve. No more efficacious than placebo in infants 6–24 months
Zafirlukast	10 mg tablet	10 mg bid (7–11 years of age)	For zafirlukast, administration with meals decreases bioavailability; take at least 1 hour before or 2 hours after meals. Monitor for signs and symptoms of hepatic dysfunction.
Methylxanthines			
Theophylline	Liquids, sustained-release tablets, and capsules	Starting dose 10 mg/kg/day; usual maximum: 16 mg/kg/day	Adjust dosage to achieve serum concentration of 5–15 mcg/mL at steady state (at least 48 hours on same dosage). Due to wide interpatient variability in theophylline metabolic clearance, routine serum theophylline level monitoring is essential.

DPI = dry-powder inhaler; EIB = exercise-induced bronchospasm; HFA = hydrofluoroalkane (inhaler propellant); MDI = metered-dose inhaler

Adapted from: National Heart, Lung, and Blood Institute. National Asthma Education and Prevention Program Expert Panel Report 3: Guidelines for the Diagnosis and Management of Asthma Full Report 2007. http://www.nhlbi.nih.gov/guidelines/asthma/asthsumm.pdf. Accessed April 2, 2009.

TABLE 9.4 Levels of Asthma Control and Severity

Intermittent Asthma	*Persistent Asthma: Daily Medication* **Consultation should be considered at Step 2* **An asthma specialist should be consulted if Step 3 care or higher is required*					
Step 1	**Step 2**	**Step 3**	**Step 4**	**Step 5**	**Step 6**	Patient education and environmental control should be assessed at each step.
Preferred:	Preferred:	Preferred:	Preferred:	Preferred:	Preferred:	
SABA PRN	low-dose ICS Alternative: Cromolyn or montelukast	medium-dose ICS	medium-dose ICS + either LABA or montelukast	high-dose ICS + either LABA or montelukast	high-dose ICS + either LABA or montelukast Oral systemic corticosteroids	

Notes: Step 1 is applicable to intermittent asthma. If a child is identified as having persistent asthma, Steps 2–6 are applicable.

Step up therapy as needed (first check adherence, inhaler technique, and environmental control).

Step down therapy when possible (and asthma is well controlled at least 3 months).

Quick-relief medication for all patients

SABA as needed for symptoms. Intensity of treatment depends on severity of symptoms.

With viral respiratory infection: SABA q 4–6 hours up to 24 hours (longer with physician consult). Consider short course of oral systemic corticosteroids if exacerbation is severe or patient has history of previous severe exacerbations.

Caution: frequent use of SABA may indicate the need to step up treatment. See text for recommendations on initiating daily long-term-control therapy.

ICS = inhaled corticosteroid; LABA = inhaled long-acting beta$_2$-agonist; SABA = inhaled short-acting beta$_2$-agonist (alphabetical order is used when more than one treatment option is listed within either preferred or alternative therapy)

Notes: The stepwise approach is meant to assist, not replace, the clinical decision making required to meet individual patient needs.

If alternative treatment is used and response is inadequate, discontinue it and use the preferred treatment before stepping up.

If clear benefit is not observed within 4–6 weeks and patient/family medication technique and adherence are satisfactory, consider adjusting therapy or alternative diagnosis.

Studies on children 0–4 years of age are limited. Step 2 preferred therapy is based on Evidence A. All other recommendations are based on expert opinion and extrapolation from studies in older children.

Adapted from: National Heart, Lung, and Blood Institute. National Asthma Education and Prevention Program Expert Panel Report 3: Guidelines for the Diagnosis and Management of Asthma Full Report 2007. http://www.nhlbi.nih.gov/guidelines/asthma/asthsumm.pdf. Accessed April 2, 2009.

Step 2 Care for Children 5–11 Years of Age

Daily long-term control medication accompanied by the availability of reliever medications is the recommended therapy for persistent asthma. The dosage of the medication should be adjusted to utilize the minimal dose possible to achieve and maintain control. The guidelines recognize that a course of oral systemic corticosteroids may be warranted to gain more rapid control of asthma in children who have experienced an exacerbation. Alternative controller medications that could be considered include (listed in alphabetical order) cromolyn, LTRAs, nedocromil, and theophylline.[1]

Step 3 Care for Children 5–11 Years of Age

For children whose asthma is not controlled by Step 2, low-dose ICS plus the addition of adjunctive therapy or medium-dose ICS is recommended. The adjunctive therapies that may be considered are: (listed in alphabetical order) LABAs, LTRAs, or, with appropriate monitoring, theophylline. Increasing the dose of the ICS to a medium level or adding a LABA are the preferred steps according to the guidelines.[1] See Table 9.5 for comparative daily doses of corticosteroids in children.

TABLE 9.5 Estimated Comparative Daily Dosages for Inhaled Corticosteroids in Children 5–11 Years of Age

Drug	*Low Daily Dose*	*Medium Daily Dose*	*High Daily Dose*
Beclomethasone HFA 40 or 80 mcg/puff	80–160 mcg	> 160–320 mcg	> 320 mcg
Budesonide DPI 90, 180, or 200 mcg/inhalation	180–400 mcg	> 400–800 mcg	> 800 mcg
Budesonide inhaled Inhalation suspension for nebulization (child dose)	0.5 mg	1.0 mg	2.0 mg
Flunisolide 250 mcg/puff	500–750 mcg	1000–1250 mcg	> 1250 mcg
Flunisolide HFA 80 mcg/puff	160 mcg	320 mcg	≥ 640 mcg
Fluticasone HFA/MDI: 44, 110, or 220 mcg/puff	88–176 mcg	> 176–352 mcg	> 352 mcg
DPI: 50, 100, or 250 mcg/inhalation	100–200 mcg	> 200–400 mcg	> 400 mcg

TABLE 9.5 Estimated Comparative Daily Dosages for Inhaled Corticosteroids in Children 5–11 Years of Age *(Cont.)*

Drug	*Low Daily Dose*	*Medium Daily Dose*	*High Daily Dose*
Mometasone DPI 200 mcg/inhalation	NA	NA	NA
Triamcinolone Acetonide 75 mcg/puff	300–600 mcg	> 600–900 mcg	> 900 mcg

HFA = hydrofluoroalkane; NA = not approved and/or no data available for this age group

Notes: The most important determinant of appropriate dosing is the clinician's judgment of the patient's response to therapy. The clinician must monitor the patient's response to several clinical parameters and adjust the dose accordingly. The stepwise approach to therapy emphasizes that once control of asthma is achieved, the dose of medication should be carefully titrated to the minimum dose required to maintain control, thus reducing the potential for adverse effect.

Some doses may be outside package labeling, especially in the high-dose range. Budesonide nebulizer suspension is the only ICS with FDA-approved labeling for children < 4 years of age.

Metered-dose inhaler (MDI) dosages are expressed as the actuator dose (the amount of the drug leaving the actuator and delivered to the patient), which is the labeling required in the United States. This is different from the dosage expressed as the valve dose (the amount of drug leaving the valve, not all of which is available to the patient), which is used in many European countries and in some scientific literature. Dry-powder inhaler (DPI) doses are expressed as the amount of drug in the inhaler following activation.

For children < 4 years of age: the safety and efficacy of ICSs in children < 1 year have not been established. Children < 4 years of age generally require delivery of ICS (budesonide and fluticasone HFA) through a face mask that should fit snugly over nose and mouth and avoid nebulizing in the eyes. Wash face after each treatment to prevent local corticosteroid side effects. For budesonide, the dose may be administered 1–3 times daily. Budesonide suspension is compatible with albuterol, ipratropium, and levalbuterol nebulizer solutions in the same nebulizer. Use only jet nebulizers, as ultrasonic nebulizers are ineffective for suspensions.

For fluticasone HFA, the dose should be divided 2 times daily; the low dose for children < 4 years is higher than for children 5–11 years of age due to lower dose delivered with face mask and data on efficacy in young children.

Adapted from: National Heart, Lung, and Blood Institute. National Asthma Education and Prevention Program Expert Panel Report 3: Guidelines for the Diagnosis and Management of Asthma Full Report 2007. http://www.nhlbi.nih.gov/guidelines/asthma/asthsumm.pdf. Accessed April 2, 2009.

Step 4 Care for Children 5–11 Years of Age

The use of a medium-dose ICS and LABA is the preferred Step 4 treatment for children 5–11 years of age. Alternative, but not preferred, therapy includes the addition of either an LTRA or theophylline to a medium-dose ICS regimen.

TABLE 9.6 Long-Term Oral Systemic Corticosteroid Management

Use the lowest possible dose to achieve control.
Monitor patients closely for adverse effects.
Reduce oral systemic corticosteroids as soon as control as achieved.
Recommend consultation with an asthma specialist.

Step 5 Care for Children 5–11 Years of Age

The utilization of high-dose ICS and LABA is the preferred treatment at Step 5. Alternative add-on therapy at this level includes LTRA or theophylline, though these add-on therapies are not the preferred treatment.[1]

Step 6 Care for Children 5–11 Years of Age

For children whose asthma continues to be uncontrolled, high-dose ICS, LABA, and oral systemic corticosteroids long term is the preferred treatment. Add-on treatments with either an LTRA or theophylline and oral systemic corticosteroids may be considered, but are not the preferred therapy. A 2-week course of oral corticosteroids to confirm clinical reversibility and an effective response to therapy should be considered before starting long-term prednisone therapy. Utilization of pulmonary function studies to assess response to oral corticosteroid therapy is recommended at Step 6. If the child's response to therapy is poor, reassessment to verify the diagnosis as asthma is recommended. See Table 9.6 for considerations when using long-term corticosteroid therapy.

Adjusting Therapy

Adjusting Inhaled Corticosteroids

> The dose of ICS may be reduced about 25%–50% every 3 months to the lowest dose possible that is required to maintain control.

Treatment decisions and medication dosages should be based on the level of asthma control that has been achieved. Therapy should be stepped up or down as needed to maintain control using the lowest dosages possible of medication. Table 9.7 can assist in assessing the level of asthma control.

TABLE 9.7 Assessing Asthma Control in Children Ages 5–11 Years After Therapy Has Been Started

Components of Control		*Classification of Asthma Control (5–11 years of age)*		
		Well controlled	*Not well controlled*	*Very poorly controlled*
Impairment	Symptoms	≤ 2 days per week but not more than once on each day	> 2 days/week or multiple times on ≤ 2 days per week	Throughout the day
	Nighttime awakenings	≤ 1×/month	≥ 2×/month	≥ 2×/week
	Interference with normal activity	None	Some limitation	Extremely limited
	Short-acting beta$_2$-agonist use for symptom control (not for prevention of EIB)	≤ 2 days per week	> 2 days per week	Several times per day
	Lung function			
	FEV_1 or peak flow	> 80% predicted/ personal best	60%–80% predicted/ personal best	< 60% predicted/ personal best
	FEV_1 /FVC	> 80%	75%–80%	< 75%
Risk	Exacerbations requiring oral systemic corticosteroids	0–1×/year	≥ 2×/year (see note)	
		Consider severity and interval since last exacerbation.		
	Reduction in lung growth	Evaluation requires long-term follow-up.		
	Treatment-related adverse effects	Medication side effects can vary in intensity from none to very troublesome and worrisome.		
		The level of intensity does not correlate to specific levels of control but should be considered in the overall assessment of risk.		

TABLE 9.7 Assessing Asthma Control in Children Ages 5–11 Years After Therapy Has Been Started

	Classification of Asthma Control (5–11 years of age)		
Components of Control	*Well controlled*	*Not well controlled*	*Very poorly controlled*
Recommended action for treatment (see for the following treatment steps)	Maintain current step. Regular follow-up every 1–6 months. Consider step down if well controlled for at least 3 months.	Step up at least 1 step and reevaluate in 2–6 weeks. For side effects consider alternative treatment options.	Consider short course of oral systemic corticosteroids. Step up 1–2 steps and reevaluate in 2 weeks. For side effects, consider alternative treatment options.

EIB = exercise-induced bronchospasm; FEV_1 = forced expiratory volume in 1 second; FVC = forced vital capacity

Notes: The stepwise approach is meant to assist, not replace, the clinical decision making required to meet individual patient needs.

The level of control is based on the most severe impairment or risk category. Assess impairment domain by patient's/caregiver's recall of previous 2–4 weeks and by spirometry/or peak flow measures. Symptom assessment for longer periods should reflect a global assessment such as inquiring whether the patient's asthma is better or worse since the last visit.

At present, there are inadequate data to correspond frequencies of exacerbations with different levels of asthma control. In general, more frequent and intense exacerbations (e.g., requiring urgent, unscheduled care, hospitalization, or ICU admission) indicate poorer disease control. For treatment purposes, patients who had ≥ 2 exacerbations requiring oral systemic corticosteroids in the past year may be considered the same as patients who have persistent asthma, even in the absence of impairment levels consistent with persistent asthma.

Before considering a step up in therapy:

- Review adherence to medications, inhaler technique, environmental control, and comorbid conditions.
- If alternative treatment option was used in a step, discontinue it and use preferred treatment for that step.

Adapted from: National Heart, Lung, and Blood Institute. National Asthma Education and Prevention Program Expert Panel Report 3: Guidelines for the Diagnosis and Management of Asthma Full Report 2007. http://www.nhlbi.nih.gov/guidelines/asthma/asthsumm.pdf. Accessed April 2, 2009.

Follow-Up Visits

Regular follow-up is essential to good asthma management. Depending on the level of control, follow-up at 1- to 6-month intervals is appropriate. If treatment is being stepped up or down, a 3-month follow-up should be considered. During these follow-up visits asthma control should be reassessed, adjustments made, and the written asthma action plan reviewed and updated as needed. It is a good idea to include children as much as possible in the development of their action plan. Patient medication technique should also be reviewed.

Back to School

A written asthma action plan should be developed and provided to the child's school and any after school activity they may participate in. Each school district is different and may require additional signatures or forms to permit the child's asthma medication to be used and/or carried on campus. Even though the asthma action plan and the back-to-school plan have been provided to the school, it is a good idea to follow up with the school nurse to insure that he/she is aware of the child's condition. Sports and physical activities should not be limited by the child's asthma. Specific instructions should be included if there are any limitation to the child's activity levels and what steps should be taken if they experience symptoms.

References

1. National Heart, Lung, and Blood Institute. National Asthma Education and Prevention Program Expert Panel Report 3: Guidelines for the Diagnosis and Management of Asthma Full Report 2007. http://www.nhlbi.nih.gov/guidelines/asthma/asthsumm.pdf. Accessed April 2, 2009.
2. Agertoft L, Pedersen S. Effects of long-term treatment with an inhaled corticosteroid on growth and pulmonary function in asthmatic children. *Respir Med.* 1994;88(5):373–81.

10

Managing Asthma in Youths ≥ 12 Years of Age and Adults

LEARNING OBJECTIVES

- Discuss stepwise management for the control of asthma therapy in youths ≥ 12 years of age and adults.
- Review the management differences between intermittent and persistent asthma.
- Identify the recommended medication dosages for the treatment of asthma in youths ≥ 12 years of age and adults.

KEY WORDS

stepwise management
asthma action plan
components of severity
classification of asthma severity

Introduction

The goal of asthma therapy for youth ≥ 12 years of age and adults is to maintain control of asthma with the least amount of medication and minimal risk for adverse effects. The stepwise approach coupled with a written asthma action plan is recommended for achieving and maintaining control.

Selecting Initial Therapy

When selecting initial therapy, the individual's asthma severity should be assessed and used as the guide for determining the appropriate treatment. Table 10.1 is useful for assessing initial therapy.

TABLE 10.1 Assessing Asthma Control and Starting Therapy in Youths ≥ 12 Years of Age and Adults

Components of Severity		*Classification of Asthma Severity in Youths ≥ 12 Years of Age and Adults*			
			Persistent		
		Intermittent	*Mild*	*Moderate*	*Severe*
Impairment Normal FEV_1/FVC: 8–19 years of age: 85% 20–39 years of age: 80% 40–59 years of age: 75% 60–80 years of age: 70%	**Symptoms**	≤ 2 days per week	> 2 days per week but not daily	Daily	Throughout the day
	Nighttime awakenings	2×/month	3×/month	1×/week but not nightly	Often (7×/week)
	Short-acting $beta_2$-agonist use for symptom control (not for prevention of EIB)	≤ 2 days per week	> 2 days per week but not daily, and not more than 1× on any day	Daily	Several times per day
	Interference with normal activity	None	Minor limitation	Some limitation	Extremely limited
	Lung function	Normal FEV_1 between exacerbations FEV_1 > 80% Predicted FEV_1/FVC normal	FEV_1 > 80% Predicted FEV_1/FVC normal	FEV_1 > 60% but < 80% predicted FEV_1/FVC reduced 5%	FEV_1 < 60% Predicted FEV_1/FVC reduced > 5%
Risk impairment	Exacerbations requiring oral systemic corticosteroids	0–1×/year (see note)	≤ 2×/year (see note)		
		Consider severity and interval since last exacerbation. Frequency and severity may fluctuate over time for patients in any severity category. Relative annual risk of exacerbations may be related to FEV_1.			

(continues)

TABLE 10.1 Assessing Asthma Control and Starting Therapy in Youths ≥ 12 Years of Age and Adults

	Classification of Asthma Severity in Youths ≥ 12 Years of Age and Adults			
		Persistent		
Components of Severity	*Intermittent*	*Mild*	*Moderate*	*Severe*
Recommended step initiating therapy (see the following detailed treatment steps)	Step 1	Step 2	Step 3 Medium-dose ICS option and consider short course of oral systemic corticosteroids	Step 3 Medium-dose ICS option, or Step 4 and consider short course of oral systemic corticosteroids
	In 2–6 weeks, evaluate level of asthma control that is achieved and adjust therapy accordingly.			

FEV_1 = forced expiratory volume in 1 second; FVC = forced vital capacity; ICU = intensive care unit

Notes: The stepwise approach is meant to assist, not replace, the clinical decision making required to meet individual patient needs.

Level of severity is determined by assessment of both impairment and risk. Assess impairment domain by patient's/caregiver's recall of previous 2–4 weeks and spirometry. Assign severity to the most severe category in which any feature occurs.

At present, there are inadequate data to correspond frequencies of exacerbations with different levels of asthma severity. In general, more frequent and intense exacerbations (e.g., requiring urgent, unscheduled care, hospitalization, or ICU admission) indicate greater underlying disease severity. For treatment purposes, patients who had ≥ 2 exacerbations requiring oral systemic corticosteroids in the past year may be considered the same as patients who have persistent asthma, even in the absence of impairment levels consistent with persistent asthma.

Adapted from: National Heart, Lung, and Blood Institute. National Asthma Education and Prevention Program Expert Panel Report 3: Guidelines for the Diagnosis and Management of Asthma Full Report 2007. http://www.nhlbi.nih.gov/guidelines/asthma/asthsumm.pdf. Accessed April 2, 2009.

It should be noted that some individuals who have moderate or severe asthma that frequently interferes with their sleep or normal activity may benefit from a course of oral corticosteroids to gain control of their asthma.[1] Once the individuals' asthma has been controlled, a stepwise management plan should be used to guide their treatment decisions.

Stepwise Management

A stepwise management plan can guide clinicians in their progressive stepping up or stepping down of therapy as needed. The steps are based on the severity of asthma at the time, and it is intended that the lowest dose possible of medication be used when managing the individual's asthma. Step 1 is applicable to intermittent asthma. Steps 2–6 are applicable to persistent asthma. Table 10.2 can assist in determining the level of asthma control and severity.

Step 1 Care

Intermittent Asthma

Step 1 establishes the baseline therapy that is to be used by all asthmatics. Step 1 includes the use of reliever medications and SABAs. The recommended therapy for intermittent asthma is a reliever medication, specifically a SABA, taken as needed to treat symptoms. These medications can be continued on an as-needed basis to manage symptoms. If SABAs are needed for quick relief more than 2 days a week (excluding the use for exacerbations caused by viral infections and for EIB), the individual should be considered as having persistent asthma. Individuals with intermittent asthma may experience sudden, severe, and life-threatening exacerbations, thus having a detailed asthma action plan to identify their symptoms and respond accordingly is important. This plan should include indicators/signs of worsening asthma symptoms and PEF measurements, specific recommendations for reliever medications, and early administration of a course of oral systemic corticosteroids. If an individual has had two or more exacerbations requiring oral corticosteroids in the past year, they should be considered as having persistent asthma.

Reliever medication should be selected at a level that achieves asthma control with the lowest dose needed.[1] The recommended dosages for reliever medication in youths ≥ 12 years of age and adults are shown in Table 10.3.

Persistent Asthma

Individuals with persistent asthma should be treated with daily long-term control medication that has anti-inflammatory capabilities. Inhaled corticosteroids are the medication of choice as a controller, though reliever medication (SABAs) must be available as needed to relieve symptoms in all

TABLE 10.2 Determining the Level of Asthma Control and Severity

Intermittent Asthma	*Persistent Asthma: Daily Medication* **Consult with asthma specialist if Step 4 care or higher is required.* **Consider consultation at Step 3.*					
Step 1	**Step 2**	**Step 3**	**Step 4**	**Step 5**	**Step 6**	Patient education, environmental control, and management of comorbidities should be assessed at each step.
Preferred: SABA PRN	Preferred: Low-dose ICS Alternative: cromolyn, LTRA, nedocromil, or theophylline	Preferred: Low-dose ICS + LABA or medium-dose ICS Alternative: low-dose ICS + either LTRA, theophylline, or zileuton	Preferred: Medium-dose ICS + LABA Alternative: medium-dose ICS + either LTRA, theophylline, or zileuton	Preferred: High-dose ICS + LABA and consider omalizumab for patients who have allergies	Preferred: ICS + LABA + oral corticosteroid and consider omalizumab for patients who have allergies	

Steps 2–4: consider subcutaneous allergen immunotherapy for patients who have allergic asthma (see notes).

Quick-relief medication for all patients

SABA as needed for symptoms. Intensity of treatment depends on severity of symptoms: up to 3 treatments at 20-minute intervals as needed. Short course of oral systemic corticosteroids may be needed.

Use of SABA > 2 days a week for symptom relief (not for prevention of EIB) generally indicates inadequate control and the need to step up treatment.

EIB = exercise-induced bronchospasm; ICS = inhaled corticosteroids; LABA = long-acting inhaled beta$_2$-agonist; LTRA = leukotriene receptor antagonist; SABA = inhaled short-acting beta$_2$-agonist (alphabetical order is used when more than one treatment option is listed within either preferred or alternative therapy)

Notes: The stepwise approach is meant to assist, not replace, the clinical decision making required to meet individual patient needs.

If alternative treatment is used and response is inadequate, discontinue it and use the preferred treatment before stepping up.

Zileuton is a less desirable alternative due to limited studies as adjunctive therapy and the need to monitor liver function. Theophylline requires monitoring of serum concentration levels.

In Step 6, before oral systemic corticosteroids are introduced, a trial of high-dose ICS, LABA, and either LTRA, theophylline, or zileuton may be considered, although this approach has not been studied in clinical trials.

Steps 1, 2, and 3 preferred therapies are based on Evidence A; Step 3 alternative therapy is based on Evidence A for LTRA, Evidence B for theophylline, and Evidence D for zileuton. Step 4 preferred therapy is based on Evidence B, and alternative therapy is based on Evidence B for LTRA and theophylline, and Evidence D for zileuton. Step 5 preferred therapy is based on Evidence B. Step 6 preferred therapy is based on Evidence B for omalizumab.

Immunotherapy for Steps 2–4 is based on Evidence B for house dust mites, animal danders, and pollens; evidence is weak or lacking for molds and cockroaches. Evidence is strongest for immunotherapy with single allergens. The role of allergy in asthma is greater in children than in adults.

Clinicians who administer immunotherapy or omalizumab should be prepared and equipped to identify and treat anaphylaxis should it occur.

Adapted from: National Heart, Lung, and Blood Institute. National Asthma Education and Prevention Program Expert Panel Report 3: Guidelines for the Diagnosis and Management of Asthma Full Report 2007. http://www.nhlbi.nih.gov/guidelines/asthma/asthsumm.pdf. Accessed April 2, 2009.

TABLE 10.3 Usual Dosages for Reliever Medication in Youths ≥ 12 Years of Age and Adults

Inhaled Short-Acting Beta$_2$-Agonists (SABAs)			
Medication	*Formulation*	*5–11 years*	*Comments*
	MDI		An increasing use or lack of expected effect indicates diminished control of asthma. Not recommended for long-term daily treatment. Regular use exceeding 2 days per week for symptom control (not prevention of EIB) indicates the need to step up therapy. Differences in potency exist, but all products are essentially comparable on a per puff basis. May double usual dose for mild exacerbations. Should prime the inhaler by releasing four actuations prior to use. Periodically clean HFA activator, as drug may block/plug orifice. Nonselective agents (i.e., epinephrine, isoproterenol, metaproterenol) are not recommended due to their potential for excessive cardiac stimulation, especially in high doses.
Albuterol CFC	90 mcg/puff, 200 puffs/canister	1–2 puffs 5 minutes before exercise 2 puffs every 4–6 hours as needed	
Albuterol HFA	90 mcg/puff, 200 puffs/canister		
Levalbuterol HFA	45 mcg/puff, 200 puffs/canister		
Pirbuterol CFC Autohaler	200 mcg/puff, 400 puffs/canister		
	Nebulizer		May mix with budesonide inhalant suspension, cromolyn, or ipratropium nebulizer solutions. May double dose for severe exacerbations.
Albuterol	0.63 mg/3 mL 1.25 mg/3 mL 2.5 mg/3 mL 5 mg/mL (0.5%)	1.25–5 mg in 3 cc of saline q 4–8 hours, as needed	

Levalbuterol (R-albuterol)	0.31 mg/3 mL 0.63 mg/3 mL 1.25 mg/0.5 mL 1.25 mg/3 mL	0.31–0.63 mg, q 8 hours, as needed	Compatible with budesonide inhalant suspension. The product is a sterile-filled, preservative-free unit dose vial.
Anticholinergics			
Ipratropium HFA	**MDI** 17 mcg/puff, 200 puffs/canister **Nebulizer** 0.25 mg/mL (0.025%)	2–3 puffs q 6 hours 0.25 mg q 6 hours	Evidence is lacking for anticholinergics producing added benefit to beta$_2$-agonists in long-term control asthma therapy.
Ipratropium with albuterol	**MDI** 18 mcg/puff of ipratropium bromide and 90 mcg/puff of albuterol 200 puffs/canister **Nebulizer**	2–3 puffs q 6 hours 3 mL q 4–6 hours	Contains EDTA to prevent discoloration of the solution. This additive does not induce bronchospasm.

(continues)

TABLE 10.3 Usual Dosages for Reliever Medication in Youths ≥ 12 Years of Age and Adults

		Inhaled Short-Acting Beta$_2$-Agonists (SABAs)	
Medication	*Formulation*	*5–11 years*	*Comments*
Systemic corticosteroids			
Methyl-prednisolone	2, 4, 6, 8, 16, 32 mg tablets	Short course "burst": 40–60 mg/day as single or 2 divided doses for 3–10 days	Short courses or "bursts" are effective for establishing control when initiating therapy or during a period of gradual deterioration. The burst should be continued until symptoms resolve and the PEF is at least 80% of personal best. This usually requires 3–10 days but may require longer. There is no evidence that tapering the dose following improvement prevents relapse.
Prednisolone	5 mg tablets, 5 mg/5 cc, 15 mg/5 cc		
Prednisone	1, 2.5, 5, 10, 20, 50 mg tablets; 5 mg/cc, 5 mg/5 cc		
Methyl-prednisolone acetate	**Repository injection** 40 mg/mL 80 mg/mL	240 mg IM once	May be used in place of a short burst of oral steroids in patients who are vomiting or if adherence is a problem.

CFC = chlorofluorocarbon; EIB = exercise-induced bronchospasm; HFA = hydrofluoroalkane; IM = intramuscular; MDI = metered-dose inhaler; PEF = peak expiratory flow

Adapted from: National Heart, Lung, and Blood Institute. National Asthma Education and Prevention Program Expert Panel Report 3: Guidelines for the Diagnosis and Management of Asthma Full Report 2007. http://www.nhlbi.nih.gov/guidelines/asthma/asthsumm.pdf. Accessed April 2, 2009.

individuals who have persistent asthma. Use of a SABA more than 2 days a week for symptom control indicates the need to step up therapy.

Seasonal Asthma

Individuals who have asthma triggered by molds or pollen and only experience seasonal exacerbations of their asthma with few symptoms the rest of the year should be considered as having persistent asthma during their trigger season and as having intermittent asthma the remainder of the time.

Step 2 Care

Long-Term Control Medications

The recommended treatment for Step 2 care is daily low-dose ICS. The alternative therapies include cromolyn, LTRA, nedocromil (Evidence A), and sustained-release theophylline. The recommended dosages for long-term controller medications in youths ≥ 12 years of age and adults are shown in Table 10.4.

Step 3 Care

Long-Term Control Medications

Individuals requiring Step 3 care should be considered for consultation with an asthma specialist. There are two acceptable preferred treatment routes at Step 3 for youths ≥ 12 years of age and adults. The first treatment route includes the addition of a LABA to the individual's low-dose ICS regimen. The second option is to continue the use of the ICS as monotherapy, but to increase the dose to a medium-dose level.[1]

Table 10.5 provides information on the dosing levels for ICS in youths ≥ 12 years of age and adults.

The alternative treatment options at Step 3 would be the addition of an LTRA, theophylline, or zileuton to the low-dose ICS treatment regimen. If one of these alternatives is used and is shown to not be effective in gaining/maintaining control, one of the two preferred Step 3 options should be tried before moving to Step 4 therapies.[1]

Step 4 Care

Long-Term Control Medications

Increasing the ICS dosage to the medium-dose range and adding a LABA is the preferred therapy at the Step 4 level. The alternative, but not preferred, therapy is the addition of either an LTRA, theophylline, or zileuton to the medium-dose ICS therapy. If one of these add-on therapies does not lead to

TABLE 10.4 Usual Dosages for Long-Term Control Medication in Youths ≥ 12 Years of Age and Adults

Dosages are provided for those products that have been approved by the FDA or have sufficient clinical trial safety and efficacy data in the appropriate age ranges to support their use.

Systemic Corticosteroids			
Medication	*Formulation*	*Youths ≥ 12 years of age and adults*	*Comments*
Methyl-prednisolone	2, 4, 8, 16, 32 mg tablets	7.5–60 mg daily in a single dose in a.m. or qod as needed for control	For long-term treatment of severe persistent asthma, administer single dose in a.m. either daily or on alternate days (alternate-day therapy may produce less adrenal suppression). Short courses or "bursts" are effective for establishing control when initiating therapy or during a period of gradual deterioration. There is no evidence that tapering the dose following improvement in symptom control and pulmonary function prevents relapse.
Prednisolone	5 mg tablets, 5 mg/5 cc, 15 mg/5 cc	Short-course "burst": to achieve control, 40–60 mg per day as single or 2 divided doses for 3–10 days	
Prednisone	1, 2.5, 5, 10, 20, 50 mg tablets; 5 mg/cc, 5 mg/5 cc		

Long-acting beta$_2$-agonists (LABAs)			
Salmeterol	**DPI** 50 mcg blister	1 blister q 12 hours	Should not be used for symptom relief or exacerbations. Use with ICS.
Formoterol	**DPI** 12 mcg single-use capsule	1 capsule q 12 hours	Decreased duration of protection against EIB may occur with regular use. Each capsule is for single use only; additional doses should not be administered for at least 12 hours. Capsules should be used only with the Aerolizor™ inhaler and should not be taken orally.
Combined medication			
Fluticasone/ salmeterol	**DPI** 100 mcg/50 mcg **HFA** 45 mcg/21 mcg 115 mcg/21 mcg 230 mcg/21 mcg	1 inhalation bid; dose depends on severity of asthma	100/50 DPI or 45/21 HFA for patient not controlled on low- to medium-dose ICS. 250/50 DPI or 115/21 HFA for patients not controlled on medium- to high-dose ICS.
Budesonide/ formoterol	**HFA MDI** 80 mcg/4.5 mcg 160 mcg/4.5 mcg	2 inhalations bid; dose depends on severity of asthma	80/4.5 for patients who have asthma not controlled on low- to medium-dose ICS 160/4.5 for patients who have asthma not controlled on medium- to high-dose ICS.

(continues)

TABLE 10.4 Usual Dosages for Long-Term Control Medication in Youths ≥ 12 Years of Age and Adults *(Cont.)*

		Systemic Corticosteroids	
Medication	*Formulation*	*Youths ≥ 12 years of age and adults*	*Comments*
Cromolyn/nedocromil			
Cromolyn	**MDI**	2 puffs qid	4–6 week trial may be needed to determine maximum benefit.
	0.8 mg/puff	1 ampule qid	Dose by MDI may be inadequate to affect hyperresponsiveness.
	Nebulizer		One dose before exercise or allergen exposure provides effective prophylaxis for 1–2 hours. Not as effective as inhaled beta$_2$-agonists for EIB.
	20 mg/ampule		
Nedocromil	**MDI**	2 puffs qid	Once control is achieved, the frequency of dosing may be reduced.
	1.75 mg/puff		
Leukotriene receptor antagonists (LTRAs)			
Montelukast	4 mg or 5 mg chewable tablet	10 mg qhs	Montelukast exhibits a flat dose response curve. Doses > 10 mg will not produce a greater response in adults.
	4 mg granule packets		For zafirlukast, administration with meals decreases bioavailability; take at least 1 hour before or 2 hours after meals.
Zafirlukast	10 or 20 mg tablet	40 mg daily (20 mg tablet bid)	Monitor for signs and symptoms of hepatic dysfunction.
5-Lipoxygenase inhibitor			
Zileuton	600 mg tablet	2400 mg daily (give tablets qid)	For zileuton, monitor hepatic enzymes

Methylxanthines			
Theophylline	Liquids, sustained-release tablets, and capsules	Starting dose 10 mg/kg/day up to 300 mg maximum; usual maximum 800 mg/day	Adjust dosage to achieve serum concentration of 5–15 mcg/mL at steady-state (at least 48 hours on same dosage). Due to wide interpatient variability in theophylline metabolic clearance, routine serum theophylline level monitoring is essential.
Immunomodulators			
Omalizumab	**Subcutaneous injection** 150 mg/1.2 mL following reconstitution with 1.4 mL sterile water for injection	150–375 mg SC q 2–4 weeks, depending on body weight and pretreatment serum IgE level	Do not administer more than 150 mg per injection site. Monitor for anaphylaxis for 2 hours following at least the first three injections.

DPI = dry-powder inhaler; EIB = exercise-induced bronchospasm; HFA = hydrofluoroalkane (inhaler propellant); MDI = metered-dose inhaler

TABLE 10.5 Estimated Comparative Daily Dosages for Inhaled Corticosteroids in Youths ≥ 12 Years of Age and Adults

Drug	*Low Daily Dose*	*Medium Daily Dose*	*High Daily Dose*
Beclomethasone HFA 40 or 80 mcg/puff	80–240 mcg	> 240–480 mcg	> 480 mcg
Budesonide DPI 90, 180, or 200 mcg/inhalation	180–600 mcg	> 600–1200 mcg	> 1200 mcg
Flunisolide 250 mcg/puff	500–1000 mcg	> 1000–2000 mcg	> 2000 mcg
Flunisolide HFA 80 mcg/puff	320 mcg	> 320–640 mcg	> 640 mcg
Fluticasone HFA/MDI: 44, 110, or 220 mcg/puff	88–264 mcg	> 264–440 mcg	> 440 mcg
DPI: 50, 100, or 250 mcg/inhalation	100–300 mcg	> 300–500 mcg	> 500 mcg
Mometasone DPI 200 mcg/inhalation	200 mcg	400 mcg	> 400 mcg
Triamcinolone acetonide 75 mcg/puff	300–750 mcg	> 750–1500 mcg	> 1500 mcg

DPI = dry-powder inhaler; HFA = hydrofluoroalkane; MDI = metered-dose inhaler

Notes: The most important determinant of appropriate dosing is the clinician's judgment of the patient's response to therapy. The clinician must monitor the patient's response to several clinical parameters and adjust the dose accordingly. The stepwise approach to therapy emphasizes that once control of asthma is achieved, the dose of medication should be carefully titrated to the minimum dose required to maintain control, thus reducing the potential for adverse effect.

Some doses may be outside package labeling, especially in the high-dose range.

MDI dosages are expressed as the actuator dose (the amount of the drug leaving the actuator and delivered to the patient), which is the labeling required in the United States. This is different from the dosage expressed as the valve dose (the amount of drug leaving the valve, not all of which is available to the patient), which is used in many European countries and in some scientific literature. DPI doses are expressed as the amount of drug in the inhaler following activation.

Comparative dosages are based on published comparative clinical trials. The rationale for some key comparisons is summarized as follows:

- The high dose is the dose that appears likely to be the threshold beyond which significant hypothalamic-pituitary adrenal (HPA) axis suppression is produced, and, by extrapolation, the risk is increased for other clinically significant systemic effects if used for prolonged periods of time

TABLE 10.5 Estimated Comparative Daily Dosages for Inhaled Corticosteroids in Youths ≥ 12 Years of Age and Adults *(Cont.)*

- The low- and medium-doses reflect findings from dose-ranging studies in which incremental efficacy within the low- to medium-dose ranges was established without increased systemic effect as measured by overnight cortisol excretion. The studies demonstrated a relatively flat dose-response curve for efficacy at the medium-dose range; that is, increasing the dose in the high-dose range did not significantly increase efficacy but did increase systemic effect.
- The dose for budesonide and fluticasone MDI or DPI are based on recently available comparative data. These new data, including meta-analyses, show that fluticasone requires one-half the microgram dose of budesonide DPI to achieve comparable efficacy.

Adapted from: National Heart, Lung, and Blood Institute. National Asthma Education and Prevention Program Expert Panel Report 3: Guidelines for the Diagnosis and Management of Asthma Full Report 2007. http://www.nhlbi.nih.gov/guidelines/asthma/asthsumm.pdf. Accessed April 2, 2009.

improvement in asthma control, they should be discontinued and another tried before stepping up to Step 5.

Step 5 Care

Long-Term Control Medications

The preferred treatment in Step 5 care includes the use of high-dose ICS and a LABA. Consultation with an asthma specialist is recommended for individuals at the Step 5 level. Individuals who are sensitive to relevant perennial allergens, such as dust mites, cockroaches, or animal dander, may be considered for the immunodulator, omalizumab. However, practitioners administering this therapy should be prepared and equipped for the identification and treatment of anaphylaxis should it occur. The optimal length of time that an individual receiving an omalizumab injection should be observed has not been established. Individuals should be educated on the recognition of anaphylaxis symptoms and the appropriate actions to take in the event of a reaction. It is a good idea to include this information on the written asthma action plan.

Step 6 Care

Long-Term Control Medications

If Step 5 therapy does not succeed in gaining/maintaining control of the individual's asthma, the addition of oral corticosteroids to Step 5 therapy is the preferred treatment at Step 6. See Table 10.6 for considerations when using corticosteroid therapy.

While the current U.S. guidelines make recommendations for anyone 12 years of age or older in one category, treatment choices should be made on a

TABLE 10.6 Long-Term Oral Systemic Corticosteroid Management

Use the lowest dose possible to achieve control.
Monitor patients closely for adverse effects.
Reduce oral systemic corticosteroids as soon as control is achieved.
Recommend consultation with an asthma specialist.

case-by-case basis. Some of the differences that should be considered when treating adolescents versus adults are listed in Table 10.7.

Treatment decisions for older adults may also vary. Table 10.8 discusses some of the considerations for this age group.

Adjusting Therapy

The decision to adjust an individual's asthma therapy should be based on their current level of control and with the intent that the lowest dose possible of asthma medication should be used to achieve and maintain control. Prior to increasing therapy a careful assessment of the individual's inhaler technique, adherence to therapy, and assessment of the environmental control measures for triggers that provoke their asthma is warranted. Generally, a step up of one level is sufficient to gain control of an individual's asthma. However, stepping up two steps may be considered in individuals who have very poorly controlled asthma.[1] See Table 10.9 for keys to deteriorating asthma.

If a deterioration of asthma is noted, a temporary increase in anti-inflammatory therapy such as a short course of oral prednisone may be indicated to

TABLE 10.7 Treating Adolescents/School Age Children versus Adults

The current U.S. Guidelines recommend that school-age children and adolescents follow the same basic medication guidelines as those set forth for adults.
PFTs should be performed using comparison data from the appropriate age/reference population. Children may need special training/coaching to achieve the best possible effort.
Adolescents (and younger children as appropriate) should be directly involved in developing their written asthma action plans.
A school plan should be developed and regularly updated. The plan should include instructions for identifying and managing symptoms; recommendations for long-term control medications; recommendations for the control and prevention of EIB, if appropriate; identification and avoidance of the individual's asthma triggers; and emergency contact information.

TABLE 10.8 Treating Older Adults

The U.S. guidelines recommend assessing the degree of reversible airflow obstruction to confirm the diagnosis of asthma and rule out other obstructive lung disease.

Asthma medication dosage and responses should be assessed and reviewed regularly for several reasons:

- Airway response to bronchodilators may change with age.
- Individuals with preexisting ischemic heart disease may be more sensitive to beta$_2$-agonist side effects.
- Theophylline clearance may be reduced in elderly patients.
- Systemic corticosteroids may cause confusion, agitation, and changes in glucose metabolism in older patients.
- Calcium supplements, vitamin D, and bone-sparing medications may be needed in individuals at risk for osteoporosis or low bone mineral density.

Medications taken for comorbid conditions such as nonsteroidal anti-inflammatory agents for arthritis, beta-blockers for hypertension (particularly nonselective beta-blockers), or beta-blockers found in some eye drops for glaucoma may exacerbate asthma and should be reviewed and adjusted as needed.

reestablish control. If the prednisone therapy does not control the symptoms, is only effective for a short period of time (less than 1–2 weeks), or is repeated frequently, the individual should be moved to the next higher step of care. See Table 10.10 for when to consult an asthma specialist.

Table 10.11 is useful in assessing therapy after an inhaled corticosteroid has been started.

TABLE 10.9 Characterizations of a Deterioration of Asthma

- A gradual reduction in PEF (approximately 20%)
- A failure of SABA bronchodilators to produce a sustained response
- A decrease in exercise/activity tolerance
- The development of increasing symptoms
- Nocturnal awakenings from asthma

TABLE 10.10 When an Asthma Therapist Should Be Consulted

Achieving or maintaining control of asthma is difficult

Immunotherapy or omalizumab use is being considered

Step 4 care or higher is needed

The individual has had an exacerbation requiring a hospitalization

TABLE 10.11 Assessing Asthma Control in Youths ≥ 12 Years of Age and Adults After Therapy Has Been Started

Components of Control		*Classification of Asthma Control in Youths ≥ 12 Years of Age and Adults*		
		Well controlled	*Not well controlled*	*Very poorly controlled*
Impairment	Symptoms	≤ 2 days per week	> 2 days per week	Throughout the day
	Nighttime awakenings	≤ 2×/month	1–3×/week	≥ 4×/week
	Interference with normal activity	None	Some limitation	Extremely limited
	Short-acting $beta_2$-agonist use for symptom control (not for prevention of EIB)	≤ 2 days per week	> 2 days per week	Several times per day
	Lung function			
	FEV_1 or peak flow	> 80% predicted/ personal best	60%–80% predicted/ personal best	< 60% predicted/ personal best
	Validated questionnaires			
	ATAQ	0	1–2	3–4
	ACQ	≤ 0.75*	≥ 1.5	N/A
	ACT	≥ 20	16–19	≤ 15
Risk	Exacerbations requiring oral systemic corticosteroids	0–1×/year	≥ 2×/year (see note)	
		Consider severity and interval since last exacerbation		
	Progressive loss of lung function	Evaluation requires long-term follow-up		

	Treatment-related adverse effects	Medication side effects can vary in intensity from none to very troublesome and worrisome. The level of intensity does not correlate to specific levels of control but should be considered in the overall assessment of risk.	
Recommended action for treatment (see preceding treatment steps)	Maintain current step Regular follow-up every 1–6 months Consider step down if well controlled for at least 3 months.	Step up at least one step and reevaluate in 2–6 weeks For side effects, consider alternative treatment options	Consider short course of oral systemic corticosteroids Step up one to two steps, and reevaluate in 2 weeks For side effects, consider alternative treatment options

*ACQ values of 0.76–1.4 are indeterminate regarding well-controlled asthma.

EIB = exercise-induced bronchospasm; ICU = intensive care unit

Notes: The stepwise approach is meant to assist, not replace, the clinical decision making required to meet individual patient needs.

The level of control is based on the most severe impairment or risk category. Assess impairment domain by patient's recall of previous 2–4 weeks and by spirometry or peak flow measures. Symptom assessment for longer periods should reflect a global assessment, such as inquiring whether the patient's asthma is better or worse since the last visit.

At present, there are inadequate data to correspond frequencies of exacerbations with different levels of asthma control. In general, more frequent and intense exacerbations (e.g., requiring urgent, unscheduled care, hospitalization, or ICU admission) indicate poorer disease control. For treatment purposes, patients who had ≥ 2 exacerbations requiring oral systemic corticosteroids in the past year may be considered the same as patients who have not-well-controlled asthma, even in the absence of impairment levels consistent with not-well-controlled asthma.

Validated questionnaires for the impairment domain (the questionnaires do not assess lung function or the risk domain): ATAQ = ©Asthma Therapy Assessment Questionnaire; ACQ = ©Asthma Control Questionnaire (user package may be obtained at www.qoltech.co.uk or juniper@qoltech.co.uk); ACT = Asthma Control Test™. Minimal important difference: 1.0 for the ATAQ; 0.5 for the ACQ; not determined for the ACT.

Before stepping up in therapy:

- Review adherence to medication, inhaler technique, environmental control, and comorbid conditions.
- If an alternative treatment option was used in a step, discontinue and use the preferred treatment for that step.

Adapted from: National Heart, Lung, and Blood Institute. National Asthma Education and Prevention Program Expert Panel Report 3: Guidelines for the Diagnosis and Management of Asthma Full Report 2007. http://www.nhlbi.nih.gov/guidelines/asthma/asthsumm.pdf. Accessed April 2, 2009.

Follow-Up Visits

Follow-up visits should be completed within 2–6 weeks after starting treatment. If the individual's asthma is not well controlled at these visits, their medication techniques and adherence to therapy should be assessed and they should be advanced to the next higher step of care. Once control is achieved and maintained for at least 3 months, a step down can be considered. If individuals' asthma continues to be uncontrolled their diagnosis should be reevaluated to rule out other conditions.

Viral Infections

Viral infections can trigger asthma exacerbations and be as problematic in adult asthmatics as they are in children. If the individual's symptoms are mild, a reliever medication (SABA) every 4–6 hours for 24 hours, may be sufficient to control symptoms. If the individual requires this therapy more frequently than every 6 weeks, a step up in long-term care should be considered. If the viral respiratory infection triggers a moderate to severe asthma exacerbation, a short course of systemic corticosteroids should be considered. Individuals with a history of severe exacerbations accompanying viral respiratory infections should be considered for a regimen of systemic corticosteroids at the first sign of infection.

Reference

1. National Heart, Lung, and Blood Institute. National Asthma Education and Prevention Program Expert Panel Report 3: Guidelines for the Diagnosis and Management of Asthma Full Report 2007. http://www.nhlbi.nih.gov/guidelines/asthma/asthsumm.pdf. Accessed April 2, 2009.

11

Managing Exacerbations, Mechanical Ventilation, and Special Situations (Exercise-Induced Asthma, Pregnancy, Surgery)

LEARNING OBJECTIVES

- Discuss the early intervention and prevention of exacerbations.
- Identify the age-appropriate medication dosages based on severity.
- Discuss strategies for managing mechanically ventilated asthmatic patients.
- Review the risk factors for increased mortality in asthma.

KEY WORDS

helium-oxygen ("heliox")
noninvasive ventilation
mechanical ventilation
extracorporeal life support (ECLS)
asthma discharge plan

Managing Exacerbations

Early intervention and the prevention of exacerbations are the preferred treatment strategies for any level of asthma.[1] The individual's written asthma action plan should include detailed instructions for self-management of exacerbations at home and guidelines as to when they should seek assistance, particularly in individuals who have moderate or severe persistent asthma and anyone who has a history of severe exacerbations.

This plan should include both symptoms and peak flow measures relating to their green, yellow, and red zones of care. The plan should also include information on prompt communication between the individual and their healthcare provider/emergency services in the event of any serious deterioration in their symptoms or peak flow, decreased responsiveness to SABAs, or decreased duration of medication effect. If the individual requires emergency assistance, the five steps outlined in Table 11.1 can help in managing their asthma and gaining control.

In addition, the following algorithm has been developed to assist in the management of asthmatic patients in the ED (see Figure 11.1).

Assessing Therapy

Assessing the individual's severity can help determine the appropriate level of therapy needed to gain control of their exacerbation and prevent the symptoms from progressing to a more serious level. Table 11.2 can assist in assessing asthma severity in the ED.

TABLE 11.1 Gaining Control of Asthma

1. Assess asthma severity and determine the level of therapy needed. (See the following tables for classification of asthma severity and medication dosages.)
2. Therapeutic options:
   - Oxygen to relieve hypoxemia in moderate or severe exacerbations
   - Reliever (SABA) medication to relieve airflow obstruction, with the addition of inhaled ipratropium bromide in severe cases
   - Systemic corticosteroids to decrease airway inflammation in moderate or severe asthma or for individuals who do not respond promptly and completely to a reliever medication.
   - Consideration of adjunct treatments, such as intravenous magnesium sulfate or heliox, in severe exacerbations unresponsive to the preceding therapy
3. Monitoring the individual's response to therapy with lung function parameters such as peak flow measurements and symptom scores.
4. Discharge: a detailed asthma discharge plan, instructions for medications prescribed at discharge, and for increasing medications or seeking medical care if asthma worsens; review of inhaler techniques whenever possible; and consideration of initiating ICS if appropriate.
5. Referral to follow-up asthma care within 1–4 weeks.

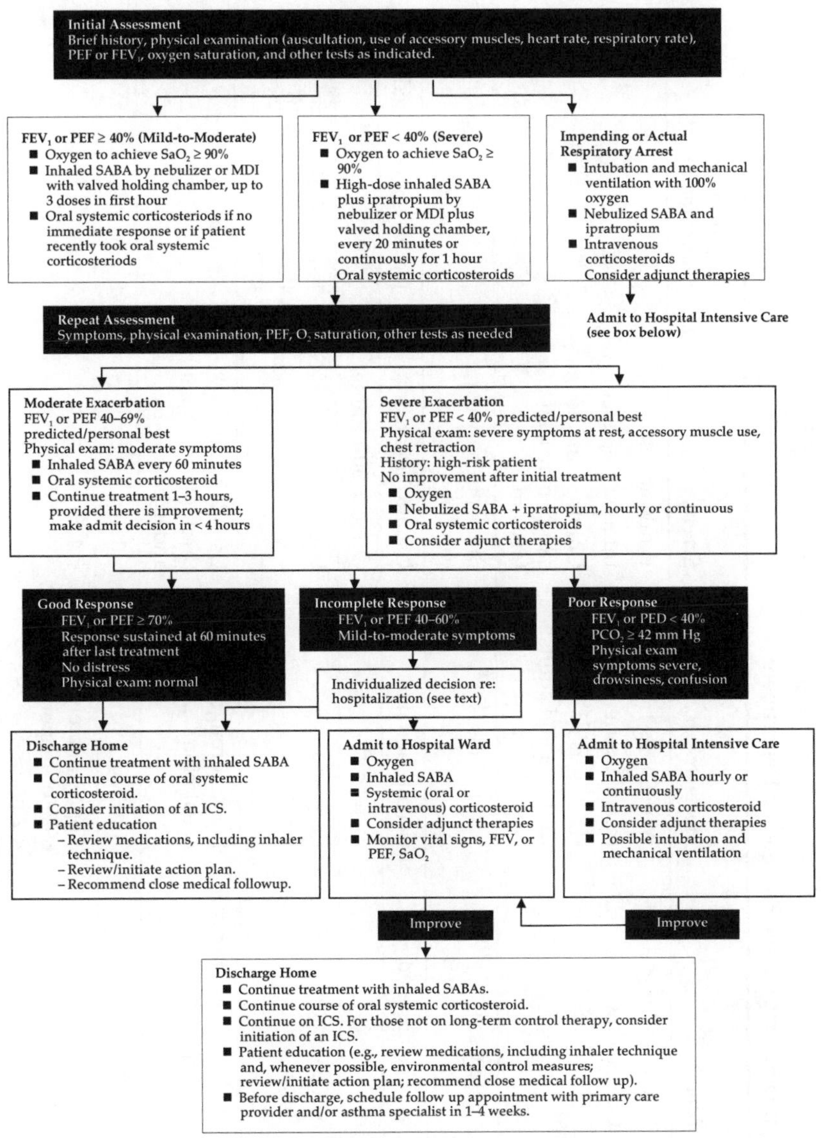

FIGURE 11.1 Management of Asthma Exacerbations: Emergency Department and Hospital-Based Care

Source: National Heart, Lung, and Blood Institute. National Asthma Education and Prevention Program Expert Panel Report 3: Guidelines for the Diagnosis and Management of Asthma Full Report 2007. http://www.nhlbi.nih.gov/guidelines/asthma/asthsumm.pdf. Accessed April 2, 2009.

TABLE 11.2 Assessing Asthma Severity in the Emergency Department

Symptoms	*Mild*	*Moderate*	*Severe*	*Respiratory Arrest/ Failure Imminent*
Breathlessness	While walking Can lie down	While at rest Infants: softer, shorter cry; difficulty feeding Children and adults: prefer to sit up	While at rest Infants: stop feeding Children and adults: sit up; may lean forward	
Talks in	Sentences	Short phrases	Breaks in between words	
Alertness	May be agitated	Usually agitated	Usually agitated	Drowsy or confused
Respiratory Rate*	Increased	Increased	Often > 30/minute	
Use of accessory muscles; suprasternal retractions	Not common at this stage	Commonly	Usually	Paradoxical thoracoabdominal movement
Wheeze	Moderate; often only end expiratory	Loud; throughout exhalation	Usually loud; throughout inhalation and exhalation	Absence of wheeze
Heart rate/minute*	< 100	100–120	> 120	Bradycardia
PEF percent predicted or percent personal best	≥ 70%	Approximately 40%–69% or response lasts < 2 hours	< 40%	< 25%

PaO_2 (on room air) (if blood gases obtained)	Normal	≥ 60 mm Hg	< 60 mm Hg: possible	
SaO_2 percent (on room air)	> 95% (test not usually necessary)	90%–95%	< 90%	
PCO_2 (if blood gases obtained)	< 42 mmHg (test not usually necessary)	< 42 mm Hg	≥ 42 mm Hg: possible respiratory failure	
Usual clinical course	Usually cared for at home Prompt relief with inhaled SABA Possible short course of oral systemic corticosteroids	Usually requires office or ED visit Relief from frequent inhaled SABA Oral systemic corticosteroids; some symptoms last for 1–2 days after treatment is begun	Usually requires ED visit and likely hospitalization Partial relief from frequent inhaled SABA Oral systemic corticosteroids; some symptoms last for > 3 days after treatment has begun Adjunctive therapies are helpful	Requires ED/ hospitalization; possible ICU Minimal or no relief from frequent inhaled SABA Intravenous corticosteroids Adjunctive therapies are helpful

*Clinicians should note that normal heart rates for infants and children differ from those of adults (see Table 11.3).

Adapted from: National Heart, Lung, and Blood Institute. National Asthma Education and Prevention Program Expert Panel Report 3: Guidelines for the Diagnosis and Management of Asthma Full Report 2007. http://www.nhlbi.nih.gov/guidelines/asthma/asthsumm.pdf. Accessed April 2, 2009.

TABLE 11.3 Normal Heart Rate and Respiratory Rates in Children

Age	*Heart Rate*	*Respiratory Rate*
2–12 months	< 160/minute	< 50/minute
1–2 years	< 120/minute	< 40/minute
2–8 years	< 110/minute	< 30/minute

Selecting the appropriate medication is dependent upon the severity of the asthma assessed. Table 11.4 can help with medication selection.

Table 11.5 details certain risk factors to note for death from asthma.

Mechanical Ventilation and Asthma

If individuals do not respond to therapy, they may require intubation and mechanical ventilation. Once intubated, weaning the asthmatic patient from mechanical ventilation can be challenging. It is important that practitioners consider mechanical ventilation a bridge to recovery, not a destination for the asthmatic. Ventilating an individual is a tool that permits the temporary restoration of gas exchange while minimizing the work of breathing until the individual can resume these functions on his/her own. For the asthmatic, gas exchange usually is not the problem. When controlling their breathing, excellent gas exchange and blood gas results suitable for textbook-weaning protocols can be achieved. The asthmatic's problem is the increased work of breathing caused by high airway resistance from the accumulation of airway secretions, constriction of airway smooth muscle, and inflammation of the airway mucosal lining. Most studies suggest that a controlled hypoventilation strategy with permissive hypercapnia is the preferred way to wean an asthmatic patient. Monitoring of the airway plateau pressure is essential to achieving this safely. Plateau pressures in the target range of 20–30 cm H_2O are usually recommended as a guide for adjustment of a minute volume that should probably start in the 90–130 mL/kg ideal body weight range. It is not uncommon for asthmatics to have intrinsic positive end-expiratory pressure (auto-PEEP) caused by their disease process, so the importance of monitoring airway pressures to optimally ventilate and prevent barotrauma cannot be stressed enough! As their airflow obstruction (airway inflammation and secretions) subside, their pressures will change and their ventilator settings should be adjusted to facilitate weaning. Clinically, the airway pressures may provide a more important indicator and a better guide for weaning these patients than the morning blood gas, providing that oxygenation and acid balance is stable.[2–4]

TABLE 11.4 Medication Dosages in the Emergency Department

Medication	*Dose for Children ≤ 12 Years of Age*	*Adult Dose*	*Comments*
Reliever medication: inhaled short-acting beta$_2$-agonists (SABAs)			
Albuterol Nebulizer (0.63 mg/3 mL, 1.25 mg/3 mL, 2.5 mg/3 mL, 5.0 mg/mL)	0.15 mg/kg (minimum dose 2.5 mg) every 20 minutes for 3 doses then 0.15–0.3 mg/kg up to 10 mg every 1–4 hours as needed, or 0.5 mg/kg/hour by continuous nebulization	2.5–5 mg every 20 minutes for 3 doses, then 2.5–10 mg every 1–4 hours as needed, or 10–15 mg/hour continuously	Only selective beta$_2$-agonists are recommended. For optimal delivery, dilute aerosols to minimum of 3 mL at gas flow of 6–8 L/min. Use large volume nebulizers for continuous administration. May mix with ipratropium nebulizer solution.
Albuterol MDI (90 mcg/puff)	4–8 puffs every 20 minutes for 3 doses, then every 1–4 hours inhalation maneuver as needed. Use VHC; add mask in children < 4 years.	4–8 puffs every 20 minutes up to 4 hours, then every 1–4 hours as needed.	In mild to moderate exacerbations, MDI plus VHC is as effective as nebulized therapy with appropriate administration technique and coaching by trained personnel.
Bitolterol Nebulizer (2 mg/mL)	See albuterol dose; thought to be half as potent as albuterol on mg basis.	See albuterol dose.	Has not been studied in severe asthma exacerbations. Do not mix with other drugs.
Bitolterol MDI (370 mcg/puff)	See albuterol MDI dose.	See albuterol MDI dose.	Has not been studied in severe asthma exacerbations.

(continues)

TABLE 11.4 Medication Dosages in the Emergency Department

Medication	*Dose for Children ≤ 12 Years of Age*	*Adult Dose*	*Comments*
Levalbuterol (R-albuterol) Nebulizer (0.63 mg/3 mL, 1.25 mg/0.5 mL 1.25 mg/3 mL)	0.075 mg/kg (minimum dose 1.25 mg) every 20 minutes for 3 doses, then 0.075–0.15 mg/kg up to 5 mg every 1–4 hours as needed.	1.25–2.5 mg every 20 minutes for 3 doses, then 1.25–5 mg every 1–4 hours as needed.	Levalbuterol administered in one-half the mg dose of albuterol provides comparable efficacy and safety. Has not been evaluated by continuous nebulization.
Levalbuterol MDI (45 mcg/puff)	See albuterol MDI dose.	See albuterol MDI dose.	
Pirbuterol MDI (200 mcg/puff)	See albuterol MDI dose; thought to be half as potent as albuterol on a mg basis.	See albuterol MDI dose.	Has not been studied in severe asthma exacerbations.
Systemic (injected) beta$_2$-agonists			
Epinephrine 1:1000 (1 mg/mL)	0.01 mg/kg up to 0.3–0.5 mg every 20 minutes for 3 doses sq.	0.3–0.5 mg every 20 minutes for 3 doses sq.	No proven advantage of systemic therapy over aerosol.
Terbutaline (1 mg/mL)	0.01 mg/kg every 20 minutes for 3 doses then every 2–6 hours as needed sq.	0.25 mg every 20 minutes for 3 doses sq.	No proven advantage of systemic therapy over aerosol.

Anticholinergics			
Ipratropium bromide Nebulizer (0.25 mg/mL)	0.25–0.5 mg every 20 minutes for 3 doses, then as needed	0.5 mg every 20 minutes for 3 doses then as needed	May mix in same nebulizer with albuterol. Should not be used as first-line therapy; should be added to SABA therapy for severe exacerbations. The addition of ipratropium has not been shown to provide further benefit once the patient is hospitalized.
Ipratropium bromide MDI (18 mcg/puff)	4–8 puffs every 20 minutes as needed up to 3 hours	8 puffs every 20 minutes as needed up to 3 hours	Should use with VHC and face mask for children < 4 years. Studies have examined ipratropium bromide MDI for up to 3 hours.
Ipratropium with albuterol Nebulizer (Each 3 mL vial contains 0.5 mg ipratropium bromide and 2.5 mg albuterol.)	1.5–3 mL every 20 minutes for 3 doses, then as needed	3 mL every 20 minutes for 3 doses, then as needed	May be used for up to 3 hours in the initial management of severe exacerbations. The addition of ipratropium to albuterol has not been shown to provide further benefit once the patient is hospitalized.
Ipratropium with albuterol MDI (Each puff contains 18 mcg ipratropium bromide and 90 mcg of albuterol.)	4–8 puffs every 20 minutes as needed up to 3 hours	8 puffs every 20 minutes as needed up to 3 hours	Should use with VHC and face mask for children < 4 years.

TABLE 11.4 Medication Dosages in the Emergency Department

Medication	*Dose for Children ≤ 12 Years of Age*	*Adult Dose*	*Comments*
Systemic corticosteroids			
Prednisone	1–2 mg/kg in 2 divided doses (maximum = 60 mg/day) until PEF is 70% of predicted or personal best	40–80 mg/day in 1 or 2 divided doses until PEF reaches 70% of predicted or personal best	For outpatient "burst therapy" use 40–60 mg in a single or 2 divided doses for total of 5–10 days in adults (children: 1–2 mg/kg/day maximum 60 mg/day for 3–10 days).
Methylprednisolone	1–2 mg/kg in 2 divided doses (maximum = 60 mg/day) until PEF is 70% of predicted or personal best	40–80 mg/day in 1 or 2 divided doses until PEF reaches 70% of predicted or personal best	For outpatient "burst therapy" use 40–60 mg in a single or 2 divided doses for total of 5–10 days in adults (children: 1–2 mg/kg/day maximum 60 mg/day for 3–10 days).
Prednisolone	1–2 mg/kg in 2 divided doses (maximum = 60 mg/day) until PEF is 70% of predicted or personal best	40–80 mg/day in 1 or 2 divided doses until PEF reaches 70% of predicted or personal best	For outpatient "burst therapy" use 40–60 mg in a single or 2 divided doses for total of 5–10 days in adults (children: 1–2 mg/kg/day maximum 60 mg/day for 3–10 days).

ED = emergency department; MDI = metered-dose inhaler; PEF = peak expiratory flow; VHC = valved holding chamber; ICS = inhaled corticosteroids

Notes: There is no known advantage for higher doses of corticosteroids in severe asthma exacerbations, nor is there any advantage for intravenous administration over oral therapy provided gastrointestinal transit time or absorption is not impaired.

The total course of systemic corticosteroids for an asthma exacerbation requiring an ED visit or hospitalization may last from 3–10 days. For corticosteroid courses of less than 1 week, there is no need to taper the dose. For slightly longer courses (e.g., up to 10 days), there probably is no need to taper, especially if patients are concurrently taking ICS.

ICS can be started at any point in the treatment of an asthma exacerbation.

Adapted from: National Heart, Lung, and Blood Institute. National Asthma Education and Prevention Program Expert Panel Report 3: Guidelines for the Diagnosis and Management of Asthma Full Report 2007. http://www.nhlbi.nih.gov/guidelines/asthma/asthsumm.pdf. Accessed April 2, 2009.

TABLE 11.5 Risk Factors for Death from Asthma

Asthma History
• Previous severe exacerbation (e.g., intubation or ICU admission for asthma)
• Two or more hospitalizations for asthma in the past year
• Three or more ED visits for asthma in the past year
• Hospitalization or ED visit for asthma in the past month
• Using > 2 canisters of SABA per month
• Difficulty perceiving asthma symptoms or severity of exacerbations
• Other risk factors: lack of a written asthma action plan, etc.
Social History
• Low socioeconomic status or inner-city residence
• Illicit drug use
• Major psychosocial problems
Comorbidities
• Cardiovascular disease
• Other chronic lung disease
• Chronic psychiatric disease

ED = emergency department; ICU = intensive care unit; SABA = short-acting beta$_2$-agonist

Adapted from: National Heart, Lung, and Blood Institute. National Asthma Education and Prevention Program Expert Panel Report 3: Guidelines for the Diagnosis and Management of Asthma Full Report 2007. http://www.nhlbi.nih.gov/guidelines/asthma/asthsumm.pdf. Accessed April 2, 2009.

Helium-Oxygen ("Heliox")

There is some data to suggest that helium-oxygen ("heliox") mixtures can benefit asthmatic patients. In theory, because the heliox has a lower density than oxygen and standard room air gas mixtures, the turbulent flow at the site of the airway obstruction is converted to a more laminar or smoother flow, hence ventilation becomes easier as airway resistance and work of breathing decrease. This smoother flow also facilitates the use of a smaller pressure gradient to deliver the same flow rate with a heliox mixture than the flow rate necessary in an oxygen/room air mixture. It should be noted that delivery of an FiO_2 higher than 40% is difficult with heliox, though there are some antidotal reports that it has been done. Practitioners should also note that there are specific monitoring requirements when using heliox and not all mechanical ventilators are equipped to deliver the mixture. Some ventilators are heliox-ready, others can be adapted. The type of ventilator being used and the software package installed on the unit will assist in determining the suitability of the ventilator for heliox delivery.[5,6]

Extracorporeal Life Support

Extracorporeal life support (ECLS) in the management of asthma patients has also been reported. The positive side is that use of ECLS alleviates the occurrence of ventilator-induced lung injury because the patients are either not intubated, or they are intubated but only minimally supported. The ECLS takes on the role of balancing the physiologic gas exchange needs, so airway resistance and work of breathing are not an issue. Most of this data for ECLS use in asthmatics is limited to case reports originating in the ED. In fairness, a large controlled trial of ECLS in asthmatics would be almost impossible to conduct due to the potential risk to the patients when other proven treatment modalities are available. In the ED setting there has been a lot of data on the effective use of noninvasive ventilation for asthmatics and this modality is usually a safer, cheaper option.[7]

Noninvasive Ventilation

Data has shown that noninvasive ventilation (NIV) is useful in preventing intubations in patients with chronic obstructive pulmonary disease.[8,9] However, there is limited data on the use of this technique in treating asthma and the current U.S. guidelines view NIV as an experimental approach for the management of severe asthma exacerbations.[1]

Special Situations

Exercise-Induced Bronchospasm/Asthma

Exercise-induced bronchospasm (EIB) should not limit an individuals' participation in vigorous activities/sports. The current U.S. guidelines recommend that an individual pretreat themselves with inhaled beta$_2$-agonists before exercise. This has been shown to prevent EIB in more than 80% of individuals and may be effective for 2–3 hours.[1] The data also shows that the use of LABAs can be protective for a period of up to 12 hours. However, the frequent and chronic use of LABAs for EIB is discouraged. Individuals using LABAs consistently for the management of EIB may have poorly controlled persistent asthma and should be evaluated for daily anti-inflammatory therapy. Cromolyn or nedocromil taken shortly before exercise is not as effective as a SABA, but may be an alternative in some individuals. Other aids to reducing EIB include wearing a mask or scarf over the mouth and nose to warm the air during cold weather and having a warm-up period prior to exercise.[1] Limiting an individual's outside exposure at times of the day when air quality levels are poor may also be useful.

Pregnancy

Pregnant women with asthma should be monitored throughout their pregnancy. Albuterol is the preferred reliever during pregnancy, and ICS are the preferred treatment for long-term inflammation control. Specifically, budesonide is the preferred ICS for pregnant women. Intranasal corticosteroids are recommended by the current U.S. guidelines for the treatment of allergic rhinitis. There is some data on the use of LTRAs in pregnancy and the guidelines state that they can be used. The recommended antihistamines are loratadine or cetirizine.[1]

Surgery

Individuals with asthma who are preparing to undergo surgery should be evaluated prior to their procedure. The anesthesiologists and surgeon should be made aware of their asthmatic condition and medication usage (particularly the use of oral systemic corticosteroids for longer than 2 weeks in the past 6 months), as well as the individual's current pulmonary function status. In some cases, a short course of oral systemic corticosteroids may be necessary to optimize lung function. The overall goal is to maximize individuals' FEV_1 or PEF so as to be as close to normal or their personal best as possible to minimize complications during and immediately after surgery.

References

1. National Heart, Lung, and Blood Institute. National Asthma Education and Prevention Program Expert Panel Report 3: Guidelines for the Diagnosis and Management of Asthma Full Report 2007. http://www.nhlbi.nih.gov/guidelines/asthma/asthsumm.pdf. Accessed April 2, 2009.
2. Leatherman JW. Mechanical Ventilation for Severe Asthma. In: Tobin MT, ed. *Principles and Practice of Mechanical Ventilation*. 2nd ed. New York: McGraw Hill; 2006.
3. Tuxen DV, Andersen MB, Scheinkestel CD. Mechanical Ventilation for Severe Asthma. In: Hall JB, Corbridge TC, Rodrigo C, Rodrigo GV, eds. *Acute Asthma: Assessment and Management*. New York: McGraw Hill; 2000.
4. Oddo M, Feihl F, Schaller MD, Perret C. Management of mechanical ventilation in acute severe asthma: practical aspects. *Intensive Care Med*. 2006;32(4):501–10.
5. Lee DL, Lee H, Chang HW, Chang AY, Lin SL, Huang YC. Heliox improves hemodynamics in mechanically ventilated patients with chronic obstructive pulmonary disease with systolic pressure variations. *Crit Care Med*. 2005; 33(5):968–73.

6. McGarvey JM, Pollack CV. Heliox in airway management. *Emerg Med Clin North Am*. 2008;26(4):905–20, viii.
7. Mikkelsen ME, Pugh ME, Hansen-Flaschen JH, Woo YJ, Sager JS. Emergency extracorporeal life support for asphyxic status asthmaticus. *Respir Care*. 2007;52(11):1525–9.
8. Medoff BD. Invasive and noninvasive ventilation in patients with asthma. *Respir Care*. 2008;53(6):740–48.
9. Seemungal TA, Hurst JR, Wedzicha JA. Exacerbation rate, health status and mortality in COPD—a review of potential interventions. *Int J Chron Obstruct Pulmon Dis*. 2009;4(1):203–23. Epub June 11, 2009.

Glossary

Activities of daily living: actions done normally in the course of daily living (e.g., brushing your hair, getting the mail, cooking dinner).

Airway hyperresponsiveness: increased sensitivity and constriction of the airways in response to an irritant.

Airway inflammation: excessive airway secretion usually followed by airway obstruction.

Airflow obstruction: increased resistance in the airways caused by an excess of secretions, narrowing of the airway, or both.

Allergen: a substance or particle that causes irritation and can cause an allergic reaction.

Anticholinergic medications: a class of medications that inhibit the parasympathetic nerve impulses by selectively blocking the binding of the neurotransmitter acetylcholine to its receptor site.

Antigen: a molecule that binds to an antibody.

Aspirin-exacerbated respiratory disease (AERD): another name for having aspirin-sensitive asthma or aspirin intolerance.

Asthma: a chronic inflammatory disease of the airways characterized by airway obstruction, inflammation, and hyperresponsiveness.

Asthma control: the degree to which asthma symptoms, functional impairments, and risks of adverse events are minimized and the goals of therapy are achieved.

Asthma control plan: a written plan to guide individuals in the management of their asthma.

Asthma prevalence: the total number of asthma cases in the population at a given time.

Atopy: the tendency to develop allergic diseases or experience an allergic reaction.

Bronchoconstriction: constriction of the airways due to the tightening of surrounding smooth muscle.

Bronchial hyperresponsiveness: bronchial constriction in response to an irritant or stimuli.

Bronchoprovocation tests: inhalation of nebulized methacholine or histamine to illicit an asthmatic response. Airway function is measured before and after the inhalation. Used to diagnose asthma (also known as a bronchial challenge test).

CD4$^+$ T cells: a type of lymphocyte (white blood cell).

Chemokines: small proteins that are involved in both acute and chronic inflammation.

Controller medication: preventive or maintenance medications usually used long term.

Corticosteroids: a class of hormones produced in the adrenal cortex.

Corticosteroid medications: medications used as controller medications in asthma. They can be taken orally, by intravenous administration, or inhaled.

Differential diagnosis: a systematic approach used to examine all possible disease states and eliminate or rule out other diagnoses until a final decision is reached.

Diffusing capacity of the lung for carbon monoxide (DLCO): the measurement of the partial pressure difference between inspired and expired carbon monoxide.

Dyspnea: shortness of breath or difficulty breathing.

Eosinophils: a type of leukocyte (white blood cell).

Exercise-induced bronchospasm (EIB): asthma that is triggered by physical activity.

Expert Panel Report 3 (EPR-3): the current asthma guidelines.

Extracorporeal life support (ECLS): mechanical ventilator support (blood/gas exchange) completed outside of the body via a mechanical device. If an extrathoracic cannulation is used it can also be called extracorporeal membrane oxygenation (ECMO), extracorporeal lung assist (ECLA), and extracorporeal CO_2 removal (ECCOR).

Forced expiratory volume in 1 second (FEV_1): maximal volume forcibly exhaled within 1 second.

Forced vital capacity (FVC): total air forcibly exhaled after maximal inhalation.

FEV_1/FVC: a calculated ratio of the proportion of the forced vital capacity exhaled in the first second.

FEF 25%–75%: measurement of the flow rates in the middle (25%–75%) of the FVC.

Flow-volume loop: a graphic representation of maximal inhalation and exhalation.

Gastroesophageal reflux disease (GERD): chronic symptoms or mucosal damage produced by the abnormal reflux/back flow from the stomach into the esophagus.

GINA: the Global Initiative for Asthma (GINA).

Granulocyte macrophage-colony stimulating factor (GM-CSF): a protein secreted by macrophages, T cells, mast cells, endothelial cells, and fibroblasts.

Green zone: eighty percent to one hundred percent of the individual's personal best or minimal symptoms of their asthma.

Helium-oxygen (heliox): a mixture of helium (He) and oxygen (O_2).

High-efficiency particulate air (HEPA) filter: a filter that can remove at least 99.97% of airborne particles 0.3 micrometers (µm) in diameter.

Hygiene hypothesis: the theory that asthma and allergies develop because of a lack of early childhood exposure to infectious diseases.

Immunoglobulin E (IgE): a class of immunoglobulins that includes the antibodies elicited by an allergic trigger.

Immunomodulators: medications or substances that weaken or modulate the activity of the immune system.

Intermittent asthma: a classification of asthma severity in which asthma symptoms occur, on average, less than twice a week.

Intercostal retractions: inward movement of the muscles between the ribs.

Interleukins: a class of proteins or cytokines that act as mediators between leukocytes.

Leukotriene modifiers: long-term control medications that operate by either blocking leukotriene synthesis through enzyme inhibition or interfere with the binding of a leukotriene to its receptor site.

Long-acting beta agonists (LABAs): a type of bronchodilator whose effects last for 12 hours or more.

Lymphocyte: a type of white blood cell.

Mast cell inhibitors: prevent the release of histamine and other proteins from the mast cells that cause asthma symptoms.

Maximum voluntary ventilation (MVV): the total volume of air that can be exhaled over a specified period of time.

Mechanical ventilation: using a device to mechanically assist or replace spontaneous breathing. It can be noninvasive, involving various types of face masks, or invasive, requiring endotracheal intubation or a tracheostomy.

Methylxanthines: a type of bronchodilator whose mechanism of action is not clearly understood.

Methacholine challenge: inhalation of nebulized methacholine or histamine to illicit an asthmatic response. Airway function is measured before and after the inhalation to diagnose asthma; also known as a bronchial challenge test or bronchoprovocation test.

Mild persistent asthma: a classification of asthma severity in which asthma symptoms occur less than twice a week.

Moderate persistent asthma: a classification of asthma severity in which asthma symptoms occur daily.

Noninvasive ventilation: mechanical ventilation that uses various types of face masks.

Obstructive sleep apnea (OSA): a sleep disorder characterized by pauses in breathing during sleep.

Pre- and postbronchodilatory testing: basic spirometry followed by a bronchodilator and then the spirometry is repeated to permit comparison.

Peak expiratory flow (PEF): the fastest rate that air can be exhaled.

Quality of life: the general well-being of individuals.

Red zone: less than 50% of individuals' personal best; severe symptoms of asthma are occurring and immediate action should be taken.

Severe persistent asthma: a classification of asthma severity in which asthma symptoms occur almost continually.

Short-acting beta agonists (SABAs): a type of bronchodilator used as a quick reliever of asthma symptoms.

Spacer device: a holding chamber that enhances the effectiveness of a metered-dose inhaler.

Spirometry: pulmonary function tests (PFTs) that measure lung function.

Stepwise therapy: a measured approach to managing asthma care.

Trigger: allergens or irritants that stimulate an asthmatic response.

Tumor necrosis factor (TNF): a cytokine involved in the inflammatory process.

Work-related/occupational asthma: airway disease triggered by a workplace irritant.

Yellow zone: fifty percent to eighty percent of the individual's personal best (or some symptoms of their asthma are occurring).

Index